Interdisciplinary perspectives on modern history

Editors
Robert Fogel and Stephan Thernstrom

A once charitable enterprise

A once charitable enterprise

Hospitals and health care in Brooklyn and New York, 1885–1915

DAVID ROSNER

Baruch College and
Mount Sinai School of Medicine
City University of New York

CAMBRIDGE UNIVERSITY PRESS

Cambridge
London   New York   New Rochelle
Melbourne   Sydney

Published by the Press Syndicate of the University of Cambridge
The Pitt Building, Trumpington Street, Cambridge CB2 1RP
32 East 57th Street, New York, NY 10022, USA
296 Beaconsfield Parade, Middle Park, Melbourne 3206, Australia

First published 1982

Printed in the United States of America

Library of Congress Cataloging in Publication Data
Rosner, David, 1947–
A once charitable enterprise.
(Interdisciplinary perspectives on modern
history)
Bibliography: p.
Includes index.
1. Hospital care – New York (N.Y.) – History.
2. Hospital and community – New York (N.Y.) –
History. 3. Hospital, Voluntary – New York
(N.Y.) – History. 4. New York (N.Y.) – Hospitals –
History. 5. Brooklyn (N.Y.) – Hospitals –
History. I. Title. II. Series.
RA982.N49R676   362.1′1′097471   81–21725
ISBN 0 521 24217 7   AACR2

Contents

Preface

This book began with a relatively simple premise: that the organization of health and hospital services was, in a variety of ways, a reflection of historically determined societal values and interests. It was my purpose to investigate these relationships and to understand how certain practices arose and how they changed over time. Of particular interest to me was the history of the relationship between patients, professionals, trustees, workers, and politicians, all of whom had different ideas and distinctly different goals at crucial moments when the modern health system was formed. To address the history of health care in any meaningful way it was necessary to understand the perspectives and interests of the different actors.

My own perspective was shaped by my experience as an administrator in New York's health system as well as by my training in the history of science and American social history at Harvard. It was this background that prompted me to use the tools of urban and social historians to analyze health policy issues of concern to health professionals. This book centers on the historical roots of distinctions in services based upon geography, income, race, and employment status – referred to as "access" and "availability" issues by planners and policy makers; the changing nature of trustee and staff relationships; and the development of new models of hospital and health care – which are often borrowed from business enterprises rather than from other social services. Hospitals have a role in shaping the life of the city through their control of land and capital. The degree to which the latter augment or undermine the primary service role of the hospital demands historical investigation.

All of these issues – class and race, professional and work relationships, politics and urban development, and business and management ideas in American institutions – have been central to the work of urban, labor, and other social historians over the past two decades. This book is aimed at integrating these general social history interests and techniques with the more traditional concerns of medical historians.

The cartoons that appear throughout the book are from the lead page of a national journal entitled *Hospital Management*. First published

vii

in 1915, this was one of the country's early hospital administration journals. It continually sought to educate its readers about modern ideas of management – through articles, news notices, and illustrations – and it advocated the adaptation of general principles of business management to the hospital. The illustrations, which appeared just after the period this book covers, indicate the growing national interest in transforming the older charity hospital into a modern, businesslike, "scientifically" managed medical enterprise. Although I focus on the arguments about paying patients, private resources, and the abandonment of charity care in New York and Brooklyn, the same arguments for the transformation of the hospital were being discussed nationally. In the late 1910s and 1920s a vigorous hospital-standardization movement began, which led to the organization, in 1951, of a national accrediting agency, the Joint Commission on the Accreditation of Hospitals (JCAH). More recently, other attempts to standardize hospital care have resulted in regulatory activities by the federal government.

As some of these illustrations indicate, the alliance between the hospital as a businesslike enterprise and the hospital as a charitable human service has been uneasy from the start. It is still a problematic relationship. The intent of this book is to remind us that, first and foremost, health care must be a human and social service. Only insofar as business methods improve the care of patients do such practices deserve society's support.

Many people aided and supported me in the writing of this book. Especially important in the development of the ideas embodied herein was Barbara Rosenkrantz, who provided constant intellectual support. Stephan Thernstrom, Gerald Markowitz, and Elizabeth Blackmar have all offered valuable comments on various sections of the work. Susan Reverby, with whom I have previously collaborated and with whom I continue to share ideas and information, deserves special thanks for her many valuable comments. Kathlyn Conway provided a critical eye and constant support during the entire time this volume was being written. Her substantial editorial skills added immeasurably to the clarity of the prose.

A number of individuals have aided me with helpful suggestions and comments regarding various aspects of the work: Harry Marks, Craig Zwerling, Richard Lewontin, Everett Mendelsohn, Roy Rosenzweig, Warren Leon, Martha Verbrugge, Harry Rosen, Charles Rosenberg, Karen Reeds, Elliott Sclar, and Robb Burlage. Also, there are others who have helped in a variety of less tangible but equally important ways: Alex and Sophie Rosner, John and Joan Conway, and Zach Rosner.

I would also like to acknowledge the substantial financial support provided to me by two organizations during my years at Harvard. The Josiah Macy Foundation supported me as a Macy Fellow in the History of Medicine and Biology for three years. During this time, I formulated many of the questions addressed in this volume. The National Center for Health Services Research of the Department of Health and Human Services (then the Department of Health, Education and Welfare) also awarded me a generous grant, from June 1976 through March 1978.

In addition, I am very grateful for the technical skills of Sally Battlon, Janis Bolster, Steve Fraser, Eleanor Hartnett, Barbara Hohol, Donna Scripture, and Betsy Smith.

New York City   David Rosner
April 1982

Introduction

"What do you mean 'no room'? If you want to [admit me] badly enough you'll find a place." This was the complaint of a Jewish immigrant to the superintendent of Mount Moriah Hospital in New York's lower East Side in 1909. Mount Moriah was a "penny hospital," supported by the "pennies" of working people who were members of the Galicia-Bokovina League, a society of Eastern European Jewish workers who had emigrated to the United States in the preceding decades. In this particular hospital the superintendent himself felt "upset that . . . many applicants [were] rejected for lack of space," because he understood that people who lived in cramped quarters would find it difficult to accept being turned away from a hospital for such a reason. "I have five children and three boarders in the same four rooms," remarked one applicant for admission. If space is tight in the hospital, the patient argued, the superintendent should "push the beds together and squeeze in another."[1]

Mount Moriah was an extremely small hospital cramped between "two adjoining tenements" and supported by the local immigrant working-class community to care for its own members. Because the administration was informal and there was relatively little hierarchy in its social relationships, patients felt confident that the superintendent would take their complaints seriously. Whereas patient care in other institutions sometimes seemed harsh and cruel, Mount Moriah's administrators had a personal relationship with their patients.[2] In the late nineteenth and early twentieth centuries, there were a number of small, idiosyncratic hospitals like Mount Moriah that were organized quickly in response to a particular need in a community. Often the trustees of these small facilities would act as personal guardians or patrons of particular patients, even to the extent of visiting them regularly to check their medical and moral progress. In some small facilities patients were expected to do cleaning and other housekeeping chores as part of their treatment and as a way of supporting the institution.[3]

Larger nineteenth-century facilities like New York Hospital or Presbyterian had more characteristics in common than did the smaller ones. Generally, these hospitals drew their support not from local

1

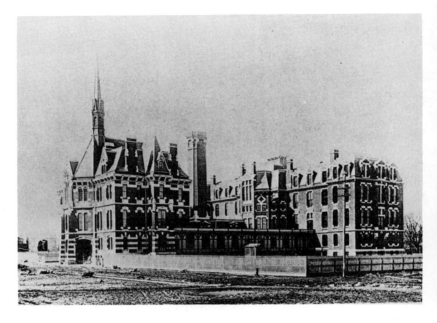

Presbyterian Hospital as it opened in 1872. In front, the churchlike administration building; in back, the ward building.

community patrons but from merchants or clergy who were important throughout the city. Because patients also came from diverse communities within the city, these hospitals were more varied in their ethnic composition. Large facilities usually had formal admissions procedures and a hierarchical bureaucratic structure, and their trustees took a paternalistic if impersonal interest in their patients. Beyond these common characteristics, however, there was great diversity among large facilities. Institutions organized by particular religious groups placed great emphasis on providing moral guidance for patients, or even converting them. Women's hospitals often provided shelter and food for pregnant unwed women and mothers for a year or longer, and children's institutions tended to resemble orphanages rather than hospitals. In this sense, both small and large hospitals reflected the idiosyncratic goals of their founders or the particular needs of their clientele much more than they conformed to any shared social definition of what a hospital should be.[4]

This volume looks at hospitals in Manhattan and Brooklyn between 1885 and 1915. During this period, the hospital system underwent a number of changes that ultimately transformed it from a series of idiosyncratic institutions to a system of acute-care facilities much like what we have today. For one thing, the number of hospitals in New York grew tremendously during the period. Whereas there were only a handful of hospitals in existence before the Civil War years, one incomplete listing compiled in the 1920s shows that at least twenty-one hospitals were organized in New York City in the 1870s, thirty-six in the 1880s, twenty-four during the 1890s, and more than forty-six in the first decade of the twentieth century. Some of the institutions that appeared between 1885 and 1915 lasted but a short time, and of these we have little record. The overwhelming majority were privately organized "charity" or "voluntary" hospitals, which, though large in number, were generally small in size. As late as the 1920s, over 37 percent of all hospitals in New York City had fewer than 100 beds.[5] The 114 independent institutions listed in an important 1924 study had an average size of under 160 beds. By the end of the period, when hospital construction began to slacken, what had started as a set of tiny local enterprises had become a major commitment: Although the hospitals were small in size, their numbers had grown to such an extent that there were six general hospital beds for every thousand residents of the city, a ratio that is close to today's figure and substantially higher than the current New York City government goal of fewer than four beds per thousand people.[6]

The number of doctors affiliated with hospitals also grew during this thirty-year period. Before the 1880s, when a hospital appointment was a closely guarded honor bestowed on particular physicians by hospital trustees, only a very restricted number of physicians had any substantial contact with hospitals. By the 1920s, however, over one-third of all physicians in New York had hospital affiliations as visiting physicians or surgeons. The locus of medical practice was clearly shifting from the home and doctor's office to the hospital.[7]

During these three decades, the hospital was also dramatically reorganized, resulting in an increase in private services and in the number of patients paying for care. In the late nineteenth century, most patients were skilled and unskilled laborers who spent their hospital stays in large open wards. Because many of them were charity cases, they were cared for in the least expensive way. Gradually, however, the number of patients paying for their care shifted the balance from ward services to private accommodations. By the late Progressive period, over a quarter of all hospital beds in New York City were in private or semiprivate rooms. By the end of this period the hospital was much more like today's institution, with relatively uniform admissions procedures; a hierarchy of doctors, nurses, and orderlies; and services that were primarily medical and were paid for by the patient.[8]

This book looks at the changes that transformed the hospital from a series of idiosyncratic community institutions into a larger, more bureaucratized system with a focus on medical treatment. It explores the forces behind many of the changes and the nature of the conflicts produced by these changes. The history of the American hospital, as far as it has been written, has been treated as part of the history of medicine and the medical profession. With the important exception of some recent work on the subject, the evolution of the modern hospital has been seen in the context of the important technical and scientific developments that transformed the medical profession during the past century.[9] Certainly, these developments had a great deal to do with changes in the hospital. Primary among the advances in the field of medicine and surgery during the middle decades of the nineteenth century was the discovery of the anesthetic properties of ether, nitrous oxide, and chloroform. Both patients and doctors became more willing to consider surgical intervention after the introduction of anesthesia. Although the number of deaths owing to postoperative infections, septicemia, or gangrene remained high, and surgery remained a technique of last resort, anesthesia did make more invasive and complex procedures possible. As a result, surgeons were able to gain the experience necessary to make surgery a more proficient and technically exact specialty.[10]

Equally as significant as the discovery of anesthesia was the development of the germ theory by such European scientists as Louis Pasteur, Joseph Lister, and Robert Koch. The germ theory spurred a search for vaccines and antitoxins to protect against or cure a variety of infectious diseases like syphilis and diphtheria. The development of the diphtheria antitoxin in the 1890s gave impetus to the search for medical cures. In the field of surgery, the understanding of the germ theory led to the development of antiseptic techniques in England and aseptic techniques in Germany, and thus made possible a reduction in the number of deaths owing to cross infections during the postoperative period. In the United States, the use of carbolic acid as an antiseptic agent and the acceptance of the need for sterility in the operating environment made it possible for surgery to advance beyond the lancing of boils, the amputation of limbs, or the setting of broken bones to the performance of more complex operations. The successful removal of the appendix was perhaps the most dramatic testament to the ability of surgeons to operate and prevent infections.[11] Certainly these changes in medical science made the hospital an increasingly attractive alternative to the home or private office. The growing hospital of the nineteenth century offered surgical rooms, equipment, and a staff of cleaners, dieticians, orderlies, and nurses who could provide constant care and attention to very sick patients.

The germ theory also ushered in a profoundly different interpretation of disease. In the nineteenth century, differences in patients' susceptibility to various conditions like consumption, venereal disease, cholera, or other infectious illnesses were often explained as matters of a patient's social situation and individual morality.[12] Within this context, medicine was a highly individualized art that demanded the utmost attention to the individual, his or her physical condition, and the social environment. By the end of the period, disease was understood in terms of the germ theory and not regarded solely as an indication of morality or social status. As a result, hospital trustees and staff came to see themselves as providers of medical treatment, not moral or social reformers.[13]

Medical historians have also explained how changes in the requirements for medical education affected the nature of the hospital. At the turn of the twentieth century the American Medical Association, the American Association of Medical Colleges, and a number of private industrial foundations worked together to raise standards for medical education. Their reform efforts culminated in the famous report written by Abraham Flexner and sponsored by the Carnegie Foundation that proposed more extensive laboratory experience and clinical exposure for students. To satisfy these demands and to gain accreditation it became necessary for medical schools to affiliate with hospitals so that they might guarantee students access to patients and clinical experience.[14]

In this book, I look at the history of the American hospital from a somewhat different perspective. Viewing the hospital as a social institution, I consider the external political, economic, and social changes that occurred during the Progressive era and that transformed the hospital. Massive immigration, political realignments, urban expansion, and a devastating economic depression placed tremendous pressure on hospitals, doctors, and other health institutions in New York during this period. For these reasons a full understanding of the changes that occurred in the hospital must take into consideration factors that profoundly affected the goals of hospital trustees, the problems to which the hospital was forced to respond, and even the nature of its patient population. Certainly changes in the nature of the hospital affected the lives of the patients and doctors who used it and in some instances even produced changes in the urban environment. The hospital was not an insular institution around which the outside world revolved, but a satellite of the larger community that reflected and was supported by that community. The growth and transformation of the hospital is part of the transformation of the American city and illustrates some of the tensions, problems, and conflicts that arose during this significant moment in American history.[15]

A social history approach encourages us to look at aspects of the history of the hospital that have previously been overlooked. For example, a small community institution like Mount Moriah provides a wealth of data for understanding the experience of its patients. Smaller institutions also provide insight into the lives of the vast majority of nineteenth- and twentieth-century physicians, who never had access to large medical centers and who spent their working lives practicing in their neighborhoods and in the wards of their local hospitals. Unfortunately, if one looks at the hospital solely in terms of great medical advances, the nature of people's experience with the hospital and the role it played in their lives can be overlooked.

A historian who considers the experience of patients and community practitioners is less likely to view the history of the hospital as one of steady progress. In fact, the concentration of care in sophisticated medical centers was often accomplished at some expense. As facilities became increasingly large and bureaucratized, and as doctors assumed more responsibilities in the hospital, care became focused less on patients' overall social and moral well-being and more on their physical and medical needs alone. Changes intended to introduce order and efficiency into the haphazard and idiosyncratic health system of the nineteenth century often resulted in a more complex, equally disordered, and sometimes less responsive system. Our modern hospital has greatly improved the quality of medical care, but in the process the hospital has lost part of its role as a community institution responsive to broader social needs that are locally identified.

My purpose is not to refute the importance of medical science in the transformation of the hospital but to examine the effect of social, economic, and political factors on the organization of the hospital and medical practice. My research focuses on institutions in Brooklyn and Manhattan at the turn of the century in the belief that the pressures on these institutions were similar to those on hospitals in other cities where industrialization and urbanization were transforming the social environment. Brooklyn's health system was composed primarily of small community-based institutions that were greatly altered and sometimes forced out of existence by external pressures. Manhattan had a greater number of large, elite medical facilities that were able to survive the pressures of change and even shape their own future. Yet the issues with which administrators and staff were forced to struggle were similar in many nineteenth-century institutions. Lay trustees and medical staffs debated whether the hospital was a place for general and varied kinds of care or a place for medical care. Private doctors who began to view the hospital as an appropriate place for treating patients had to deal with their patients' reluctance to go to a "charity" facility that had long been associated with indigency. As medicine became more specialized, community physicians found themselves competing with hospital physicians and specialists for patients. Even the long-standing system of fee-for-service payment for doctors was called into question when physicians began treating private patients in the hospital. Not until new administrative and organizational relationships among doctors, trustees, and patients were developed did the community practitioner see the hospital as a suitable place to practice. Nor were upper-class and professional people willing to use the hospital until private services and private rooms were created for them. Their entrance into the hospital often forced trustees to relinquish the stewardship role they had adopted with working-class patients and the poor.

If we look at the history of institutions, it becomes clear that significant changes in the shape of the hospital often occurred before new medical techniques were introduced. In many instances hospitals were reorganized for internal economic reasons before medical and surgical advances forced any reordering. Private and semiprivate rooms, privileges for attending and visiting physicians, full-time staff nursing, and other amenities characteristic of the modern hospital were introduced into many institutions with little regard to medical standards or necessity. In Brooklyn, for instance, trustees at one of the larger charity institutions decided to build private wings and wards well before they saw a need for an operating theater. As late as 1900, operations were performed in a hallway of the nurses' quarters.[16] In other small hospitals throughout Manhattan and Brooklyn, largely unused private services were created by trustees at a time when the most complicated surgery was little more than the binding and bandaging of surface wounds. Even the implications of the germ theory were only partially understood. As late as 1905 a committee of physicians and laymen in New York suggested that there was little reason to throw away previously used bandages: "The same material used on clean wounds for dressings should be re-washed and re-sterilized and repeatedly used." Gauze swabs and bandages, the committee added, "can be re-washed, re-sterilized and used dozens of times instead of being thrown away."[17] In the largest and most prestigious teaching hospitals, the use of the operating room was hardly commonplace during this period. At the Massachusetts General Hospital, for example, Saturday was called

"Operating Day" as late as the 1920s, and as late as 1890, most major teaching hospitals rarely had more than one operation per day.[18]

These facts lead one to consider other factors that accounted for the changes in the reorganization of health care. Chapter 1 looks at the actual physical changes in the organization of the city, the breakup or rearrangement of neighborhoods and the physical separation of the upper and middle classes from the working class. In many instances industrialization and commercialization were the giants that disrupted stable communities and undermined their systems of charity health services. Upper- and middle-class groups escaped the increasingly crowded and noisy city by moving to the developing suburbs, taking with them many doctors and abandoning the communities whose health care depended on the commitment of wealthy patrons and the presence of community practitioners. Feeling a shortage of family practitioners, unskilled laborers and other working-class people turned to those small dispensaries and hospitals within their neighborhoods which had not been forced out by realtors, merchants, and planners seeking to develop the area for commercial uses. These institutions were generally unprepared for the increased number of patients created by a depression that left thousands homeless and sick. Nor were they prepared for the increase in patients injured in accidents or suffering from diseases related to industrialism. New health-care problems were created in the suburbs, as well, by demographic changes. Doctors often had to set up new private practices or travel to see their former patients. Patients had to find new doctors or get used to the idea of traveling out of their communities to see the old ones. As populations shifted, hospitals were not necessarily located in places adjacent to or convenient for people in need. Within a few decades the community-based charity health system was under tremendous pressure to adapt to external social and demographic changes.

Chapter 2 describes how the economic depression of the 1890s, the worst of the century, began to take its toll on the health-care system. Thousands upon thousands of workers who were unemployed for extremely long periods of time turned to the charity hospital for food, shelter, and medical care. As this depression intensified, charity institutions became overcrowded and faced a serious economic crisis. The long-term rise in the costs of medical care, a decline in philanthropic donations, and rapidly growing patient rolls all threatened the very existence of charity hospitals, especially the smaller ones. Trustees of these institutions reluctantly sought new ways to gain income. Some hospitals were forced to close; some were able to survive by decreasing services; and many reluctantly began to charge patients who had previously been treated without charge or for nominal sums.

As hospital administrators began to move patients through the facilities more quickly in order to reduce costs and accommodate more
needy patients, the trustees found their traditional role as stewards for
the poor being undermined. No longer were patients present in the
hospital long enough for trustees to assume responsibility for their
social and moral improvement. Nor could pressured trustees who were
charging patients continue to see their institutions primarily as services to the poor. In fact, many charity patients came to be seen by
trustees as a burden, especially because demands for care were so high
and the need seemed so overwhelming. In the face of the seemingly
intractable poverty created by industrialization, trustees retreated
from their previous commitment to charity and sought to narrow the
scope of their hospitals.

Chapter 3 describes the evolution of a deliberate policy among hospital trustees and administrators to seek out paying patients. Trustees
converted what were called "free" wards into paying wards and private
rooms; they provided the option of private-duty nurses for those who
could pay; they introduced better food and hired nurses and orderlies
to do the maintenance chores previously done by patients. Every attempt was made to make paying patients feel that the hospital was
little else than an "invalid's hotel." To alter the public image of the
charity hospital as a place of death and suffering for the indigent or
working class, trustees began to advertise their hospital services and
their hotel-like accommodations. It soon became clear to trustees that
even these efforts were not sufficient to attract wealthy clients who
still had the option of being cared for by private family physicians in
their own homes.

The decision of trustees to turn to private family doctors for help in
bringing paying patients into the hospital is described in Chapter 4.
Trustees reasoned that if they could make an alliance with the private
doctors who controlled the therapeutic regimes of white-collar workers and of professional and other relatively wealthy patients, these
doctors might encourage their own patients to use the hospital. Doctors had long been seeking hospital appointments in order to gain
more clinical experience and to get access to patients in need of private
follow-up care. Although trustees were reluctant to admit doctors for
fear that they would assume too much control, the financial crisis left
the trustees with little choice but to admit doctors as consultants and
attending physicians. In an effort to maintain the ideals of charity
while meeting the financial needs of the hospitals, trustees sought to
maintain the former ward-based structure for nonpaying patients by
giving doctors access only to private patient beds in private pavilions
or private wards. As doctors gained clinical experience, improved their

specialty knowledge, and increased in numbers, however, they felt confident about challenging the right of lay trustees to make important policy decisions, and they began to assume more responsibility in the hospital. Antagonism developed between the doctors and the trustees, and between the doctors and the hospital superintendent. Although trustees sometimes considered that the scientific and pecuniary interests of doctors were antithetical to the goals of the older charity institution, they were forced to acknowledge the growing authority of physicians in their institutions.

While the Depression and the growing problems of hospital financing severely affected the internal workings of charity hospitals, ongoing political changes in the city also forced institutions to abandon their locally defined objectives. As Chapter 5 illustrates, by the end of the nineteenth century it was apparent to many reformers that the charity hospitals lacked a commitment to the wider needs of the city as a whole. Most specifically, many institutions seemed to ignore the growing need for emergency medical and ambulance services throughout the city, and remained concerned only with local objectives. Using as a lever a long-standing financial arrangement in which charity hospitals received funds from the city government, city comptroller Bird S. Coler pressed charity hospitals to take responsibility for the care of certain types of medical cases, along with emergency and ambulance services. Using the rhetoric and tools of Progressive reformers of the period, Coler replaced the older system of flat-grant payments, a system by which ward boss politicians had been able to secure funds for local institutions, with a per capita, per diem method for reimbursing hospitals. By centralizing decision making and setting uniform standards, Coler hoped to introduce rationality, order, and efficient business practices into informally organized charity services and to undermine the authority of local groups and Tammany Hall politicians.

Underlying Coler's reforms was the assumption that larger institutions would provide better and more efficient care. As a result, small institutions with limited bed capacity could expect funds to cover only as many patients as they had beds. Even if all their patients were charity cases reimbursable through the city, smaller institutions ended the year with less support from the city than they had obtained under the old flat-grant system.

Even as city government reforms were undermining small hospitals, the system of small charity dispensaries came under attack from the state. In the period immediately following the Depression, when these ambulatory clinics were receiving reduced incomes from the city, state inspectors set up standards and regulations that effectively crippled most of them. For the most part, the state was pressured into action by doctors who had come to see the dispensaries as competitors for those patients whose income was small. The doctors reasoned that if care were available free of charge, people would tend to abandon the services of private doctors who would charge them. Though larger dispensaries associated with hospitals managed to survive as outpatient departments, the smaller dispensaries were virtually eliminated by the combined actions of physicians, the city, and the state. As Chapter 6 illustrates, in little over a decade, nearly 100 dispensaries in New York and Brooklyn went out of existence.

Although social, economic, and political changes primarily affected small charity facilities, large hospitals also had issues to face. Chapter 7 describes the response of New York Hospital, a large Manhattan institution, to demographic changes in the developing city. New York Hospital became deeply enmeshed in a battle for control over the land upon which its mental asylum rested. As land values skyrocketed in areas of upper Manhattan in the late 1880s, realtors interested in developing the area for residential use joined with Tammany Hall politicians to attack the hospital's Bloomingdale Asylum, which was considered a major roadblock in the way of West Side development. The hospital's trustees were extremely powerful men in the city and state who fought a tremendous political battle with developers and Tammany Hall over control of the land. The Bloomingdale Asylum was ultimately forced to move from its land in Morningside Heights, but the trustees were able to guarantee that the neighborhood would remain in the hands of a Protestant elite at the very time when the growth of Harlem as a Jewish and Italian community and of the West Side as an Irish Catholic neighborhood threatened to turn the area into a working-class Catholic or Jewish community. The case of New York Hospital indicates the control that large, elite institutions were able to exert over the direction of their institutions and neighborhoods.

By the end of the Progressive era, the health care system had undergone tremendous change both internally and externally. Once the domain of local community members, the health system was increasingly influenced by forces outside the community. Economic depression, political change, and a growing belief in medical expertise brought about new standards for health-care institutions – standards that determined the shape of medical care far more than did the particular needs of the community or patient population. Locally based charity facilities were replaced by a system of health care built around the newly arising medical profession and hospital. Internally, the institution began to take its present-day form with private and semiprivate rooms, private practice medicine, and paying patients. Gone were the large wards, the atmosphere of moral reform, and the paternalism of charity care.

Though the development of the hospital as the center of care brought improved medical services, it did so at some expense. No longer could people turn to the hospital for a broad set of primary-care needs or during periods of social dislocation. The hospital had become a facility where people paid for medical services. Although changes in the hospital introduced some rationality into the haphazard older system, the hospital was rearranged but not necessarily made more orderly. In fact, the modern hospital in some sense embodies the failures of the old system as well as of the new. The disorganization of the charity system remains with us in the form of inaccessible and sometimes inappropriate facilities, often planned by those with private or provincial interests who pay little attention to gaps in the overall health system. At the same time, the modern hospital is often insensitive to the varied needs of the community for services that are not strictly medical. The relationship of hospitals to ethnic and religious communities is much weaker today than in the past. At Montefiore Hospital in the Bronx, one physician later in the twentieth century was heard to complain, "Everyone is treating the electrolytes, but who is treating the Israelites?"[19] I hope to provide part of the answer to his question in this book by looking into the social transformation of the community hospital.

1   *Health care and community change*

Nineteenth-century American life revolved around small communities and narrow personal contacts. Most Americans lived in rural villages and towns that were essentially isolated from each other, and even those who lived in the city lived in highly structured communities separated from each other by culture, ethnicity, and sometimes language. Because there were no adequate transportation and communication systems early in the century, there was little chance for relationships beyond one's immediate neighborhood. In these so-called walking cities, life revolved around the local church, school, and other small institutions. Government was a neighborhood responsibility watched over by the local ward boss, who, as part of the political machine, was able to attend to the needs of the community.[1]

A strong neighborhood focus of necessity characterized nineteenth-century medical practice as well. For much of the century, New York City was a highly congested series of neighborhoods spread between the southern tip of Manhattan and Fifty-ninth Street. Before the introduction of electric trolleys and elevated railroad lines, the horse was the major means of transportation. Although the city's gentry owned private carts and wagons for transportation, most of the working people depended upon slow and undependable horse-drawn trolleys, which had to negotiate streets that were continually "torn up, blown up or dug up"[2] for construction. In the 1860s, it was reported that "a considerable part of the working population spend a sixth part of their days on street-cars or omnibuses," and this was only for relatively limited travel in the neighborhoods below Fifty-ninth Street. The "upper part of the city [above Fifty-ninth Street] is made almost useless to persons engaged in any daily business," it was noted.[3] Unless an extreme emergency forced people to travel, most patients sought medical treatment as well as other services in their own neighborhoods.

Not only were laborers and merchants hampered by the poor system of transportation, but doctors, too, sought to avoid any great amount of travel. One physician reminisced about his early days at Metropolitan Hospital, originally a homeopathic municipal institution located on Wards Island. He estimated that the trip to the hospital from a residence in Manhattan took no less than three hours of travel time by horse and buggy and ferry.[4] Recalling the difficulties faced by younger house staff who lived at the hospital, this doctor remembered that only if someone "was fortunate enough to have friends in the village of Harlem" could he find entertainment, because "it was almost impossible for anyone . . . to go to parties or the theatre in the city and get back the same day."[5]

Some practitioners committed to certain forms of practice or in need of clinical experience or prestigious appointments were willing to travel long distances regularly. But for the vast majority of practitioners the inconvenience of travel made a local community practice extremely attractive. Only when urban redevelopment forced relocations would established practitioners leave their communities. The "elder and better established of the profession never left the older sections of the city," remembered Dr. Frederick Dearborn, "unless the encroachment of their clientele made a change necessary."[6]

Because nineteenth-century medical knowledge was inexact and professionals were not at all in agreement about the causes of illness or the proper management of disease, the choice of treatment was generally a reflection more of the customs and medical beliefs of a particular community or practitioner than of sound scientific knowledge.[7] The medicine practiced in one area of the country was often quite different from that in another. In much of rural America, lay people combined local folk custom with information gleaned from medical dictionaries and popular medical texts to form an idiosyncratic body of therapeutic practices.[8] Doctors, not yet an elite professional group, generally pursued formal medical school training and apprenticeships in their own locales. The majority of medical schools were "proprietary" or "profit-making" institutions that attracted persons from lower-middle-class and working-class backgrounds and produced practitioners of varying skill and dubious scientific training. Formal medical education was largely unregulated and nonstandardized and could vary in length, content, and structure, depending upon the demands of different areas of the country. Not only did training differ for rural and urban practitioners, but a diversity of training and background could be found among those treating different classes and ethnic groups within the population.[9]

Generally the educational requirements of various schools reflected their different medical nosologies and theoretical positions. Rural areas produced a wide variety of "sects" whose therapeutics depended mostly on herbal treatments. Thomsonians and later "eclectics" were among the various "botanists" in New England, the South, and the Midwest who incorporated local folk and Native American custom into their therapeutics.[10] In urban areas, regular practitioners, homeopaths, and a host of others with differing medical viewpoints and practices competed strongly with each other for the patronage of patients.[11] Today patients have little choice about their medical treatment, but patients in nineteenth-century America could choose among a host of practitioners and a fairly wide variety of therapies. Almost all nineteenth-century doctors were "family" or "community" practitioners who engaged in general medicine. The small number of doctors who specialized in surgery, ophthalmology, or other areas saw their specialism as tangential to their practice.[12]

The family practitioners who constituted the bulk of the profession generally lived within the communities they served and provided health services at the homes of patients or in offices in their own homes. Generally the doctor's patients lived within a few blocks of his house and were members of the church or local community organizations to which he belonged. Without question, the family doctor presided at the significant events in people's lives; he would be "fetched" for births as well as deaths, and at times would move into the patient's house for the duration of an illness.[13]

The motive for this kind of personal treatment was certainly, though not solely, the best care of the patient. Because there were a large number of loosely organized medical schools and lenient licensure requirements, there existed a surplus of practitioners who were in competition with each other for patients. Without the mid-twentieth-century options of research positions in universities or hospitals, and without highly specialized forms of practice, doctors depended entirely upon their patients for income. Consequently, competition among practitioners for patients had become fierce by the end of the century.[14] As one contemporary observer remarked, "a new doctor must create his practice out of that taken from other physicians."[15] In the absence of more formalized methods of evaluating status or competence, patients generally chose their practitioner on the basis of such criteria as familiarity, dress, courtesy, and cultivation. D. W. Cathell, a physician who wrote a widely distributed and oft-reprinted late-nineteenth-century practical guidebook for practitioners, began his volume by pointing out that "there is nothing more pitiful than to see a worthy physician deficient in these qualities, waiting year after year for a practice . . . that never come[s]."[16]

One European physician who moved to New York in the 1870s noted the significance of this uniquely American environment for the American physician's relationship to his clients. He observed that the "science and technique of practice" were less important to American doctors than were "the personal relations between physician and patient." He remarked that "physicians in America were concerned more with establishing a feeling of confidence and trust, hence comfort in patients, than were" Europeans. He ascribed this concern to the highly competitive nature of their practice and to the relatively low social and educational status of American practitioners. The "medical man had to be more modest; he had to be more circumspect, even deferential" when treating patients, even when the patients were ignorant or ill-mannered. The unique quality of highly isolated communities created a marketplace where personal relationships determined professional success.[17]

Because medical knowledge was not standardized and practitioners depended directly on their patients for a livelihood, they tended to practice in ways that were familiar to and would please their patients. It was not that doctors did not believe in their treatments; in many ways, in fact, their knowledge was only slightly more sophisticated than that of their patients. The largest group of physicians, regular practitioners, employed bleeding, cupping, purging, and other seemingly draconian measures.[18] Because illness was often equated with moral failings, treatments we view as cruel were sometimes considered an appropriate punishment for transgressions.[19] Those who rejected therapeutics often turned to other milder forms of practice like homeopathy. Widely accepted and preferred by merchants and other urban groups, homeopathy provided more elegant rationales. The lack of scientific rigor and specificity in these practices was made up for by the intimacy of the practitioner's social relationship to the patient.

Hospitals of the late-nineteenth-century city

After the Civil War, large numbers of hospitals were established in response to diverse but specific social and medical needs. Very often the elite of a community, generally local merchants, businessmen, and members of the clergy, would initiate and sponsor the formation of a hospital to serve the working class and the dependent poor. Hospitals generally differed in religious and ethnic orientation, source of financial support, size, medical orientation, and the type of service provided. Often an ethnic or religious group would establish a hospital for the dependent poor of a particular faith or neighborhood. Of the 4,500 institutions that began in the United States during the period this book examines, many bore names that identified them with a particular religious or ethnic community. Among the 130 or more hospitals that began in New York and Brooklyn, for instance, one could find religiously supported institutions like Jews Hospital, St. Vincent's Hospital, and Methodist, Lutheran, and Episcopal hospitals. German Hospital (now Lenox Hill) and Norwegian, Swedish, and Lincoln hospitals (the latter for Freedmen) all provided services for their own ethnic population. Often local benefactors would establish a hospital in response to a particular social need in the community. Children's hospitals often arose to care for orphaned children, whether in medical need or not. Maternity hospitals in working-class neighborhoods often sheltered unwed mothers in addition to providing maternity medical service. In communities with a significant number of elderly and dependent persons, local merchants often organized a home or hospital for "incurables" or for the chronically ill.[20]

Obviously many of these "hospitals" were not the large complexes we know today, but often homes that were quickly put to use when a need arose in the community. An extreme example of how quickly small hospitals were established is the Chinese Hospital of Brooklyn. As part of their missionary work among the city's newly arrived Chinese, the King's Daughters of China established a tiny five-bed hospital in Brooklyn Heights. In little over one month late in the fall of 1890, this missionary society conceived of the facility, rented space, and opened the doors to patients. "The project for a Chinese Hospital . . . owes its fruition and consummation to the 'King's Daughters of China,' " began Dr. Joseph Thoms, the superintendent of the facility, in the hospital's *First Annual Report* in 1892. "The rent being guaranteed by these ladies and acting upon their advice, I leased for the term of one year, the premises at No. 45 Hicks Street for Hospital uses, commencing our term as tenants upon November 1, 1890, at the rate of $50 per month," he continued. "Preparations were made at once to receive patients, and by the last week of the month we were ready for them, beginning with only 5 beds." On December 7, only five weeks from the time of its founding, the hospital opened.[21]

There were a number of large, publicly sponsored institutions like Bellevue Hospital in Manhattan, Kings County Hospital in Brooklyn, and Boston City Hospital in Massachusetts, and a few large charity institutions like New York Hospital, Presbyterian, and St. Luke's in New York and Massachusetts General Hospital in Boston. The public hospitals were generally organized as adjuncts to the local almshouse or prison to serve numbers of those not accommodated in the local charity facilities. Because small charity facilities often had fewer than fifty beds, they generally sent the "unworthy" poor, alcoholics, and criminals to the public hospital and served primarily the dependent poor and working-class people of their communities. The local sponsors who were the trustees of these small institutions were rarely prominent outside their particular neighborhood and often saw their commitment to the hospital as a commitment to their community or faith.[22]

Unlike its modern-day counterpart, the nineteenth-century hospital was not solely a medical facility but a facility that provided shelter, food, and care for those in need. Because the community's leaders and the middle class were generally cared for in their homes, hospitals treated those working-class people who resided in the homes of the wealthy or lacked the resources to be treated in their own homes. Methodist Hospital, located on the border of the elite, upper-middle-class neighborhood of Park Slope, reported as late as 1896 that a large number of its young female patients were domestic servants working and living in the brownstone homes of the neighborhood. "Few, when sick, are in sorer need of a hospital than they," the trustees reported. This "need" was a reflection less of a young woman's physical condition than of the social circumstances that surrounded her work and living arrangements: When women in such circumstances became ill, not only were they unable to perform the daily chores that kept the household running, but they also occupied rooms and needed care. This was experienced as a severe inconvenience by the families who supported them. "The families in which they lived feel embarrassed," the trustees pointed out, but "the work must go on and . . . another must take her place." Clearly, the servant who entered the home to perform household chores needed a place to sleep. "What can be done with the poor invalid? Her room is required. She is in the way." The tension created for the employer was minor compared to that created for the sick servant herself. The trustees pointed out that the young woman was "a burden and she knows it" and that this only increased the danger of her illness, as "the poor girl grows feverish with anxiety." The hospital provided a solution for both the wealthy family and the servant. "Her employer comes and represents the case to us," the trustees observed, "and we open the way for her to occupy a free bed." This relieved the employer of responsibility to care for her and prevented the young woman from being homeless.[23]

This situation illustrates the varied and ambiguous role of the nineteenth-century community hospital, which functioned simultaneously as a health-care facility, a social service, and an agent of social control. Admission to the hospital depended less on a patient's medical state that on the determination by a wealthy patron that the patient's physical or social circumstances made him or her an appropriate candidate for admission. "Some [patients] were at the point of death and others were apparently in robust health, their diseases . . . obscure or simply annoying," casually reported Methodist Hospital's superintendent. But one thing was sure: The patient's patron had determined that the patient was "morally worthy."[24]

The organization and sponsorship of hospitals varied as much as their functions. Lutheran Hospital, a small institution located in a new Scandinavian neighborhood of East New York, was far different in appearance from a larger hospital like Methodist. In many ways, its building was indistinguishable from the run-down one- and two-family houses scattered throughout the neighborhood. Surrounded by a picket fence and fronted by a modest lawn, the building was itself a wood-framed, three-story structure with a front porch and sloping roof. Like other houses in the neighborhood, Lutheran was home for no more than thirty patients at any given time. The hospital resembled a home on the inside as well, complete with a sitting room, rugs on the floor, and chandeliers.[25] As in any other home and as with any other "family," each household member had distinct tasks. The matron and superintendent oversaw the patients much as a mother and father might supervise their children in the house. They considered patients to be in need of training in proper morals and work habits. When physically able, patients made their beds, washed their clothes, and did other necessary tasks. As the constitution of one maternity hospital explained, "Such free patients as . . . are able, shall assist in nursing others, washing and ironing the linen and [other] services." Patients often used the hospital as a home, staying for relatively long periods of time. Through much of the century, stays of over three months were not unusual in many institutions, and the average length of stay in maternity and children's hospitals could sometimes be measured in years. Because patients lived in the institution for long periods of time, they often required social activities as well as medical supervision.[26]

Some institutions served a more direct religious function than others. The Chinese Hospital, the small facility spoken of earlier, was begun by "Christian people engaged in the work of evangelizing" immigrant Chinese. In a very real sense, its superintendents and staff measured its success more by the number of converts it made among its patients than by the number of medical cures. Medicine and morality were so closely tied together in this institution that two sets of statistics were kept: One reported on the number of patients successfully treated by what was called "Western Science," and another gave the number of patients who were converted or who "heard the Gospel" for the first time. In 1892 the hospital had a mortality rate of over 33 percent, extremely high even by nineteenth-century standards. But such statistics were easily explained away by the number of persons who arrived in the hospital in an advanced stage of illness and close to death – patients who, it was argued, had been mistreated by Chinese

HOSPITAL MANAGEMENT

June, 1917
Vol. III, No. 5

608 S. Dearborn Street, Chicago

Published in the Interest of Executives in Every Department of Hospital Work

Entered as second class matter May 14, 1917, at the post office at Chicago, Ill., under the act of March 3, 1879.

A Modern Version of The Old Woman Who Lived in a Shoe

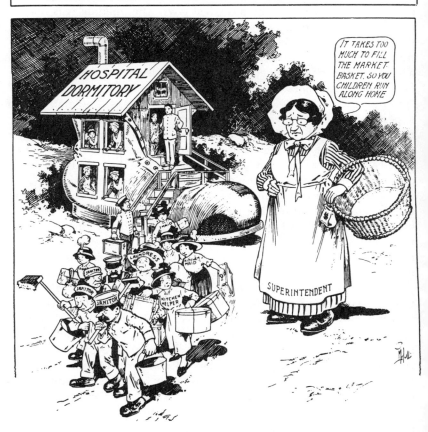

During the Progressive era the older paternalistic relationships between those who ran the institution and those who worked in it broke down. In this illustration from a 1917 issue of a new journal entitled *Hospital Management*, the hospital administrator, holding a small purse and an empty basket, sends her work force away from the hospital dormitory. Although it was a common practice to provide living accommodations to the work force during the nineteenth century, "living in-house" was gradually restricted to nurses and "house staff" physicians.

physicians. "The mortality ratio naturally looks large, but the majority of our patients are advanced cases of the incurable varieties of Phthisis, 32 of which were literally carried bodily into our Hospital," the superintendent reported. Furthermore, "with very few exceptions, these poor fellows were victims of month after month of time lost in the hands of the Chinese ignoramus called 'doctor.' "[27]

The success of the institution was only partly measured by its mortality rate, the superintendent added, as only "five [patients] were already Christians when admitted." The superintendent reported the number of conversions with a degree of detail that illuminates the significance of this role for his hospital. He noted that "three gave convincing evidence of conversion while inmates; ten had been members of Sunday schools, but the remaining 58 never before had enjoyed any opportunity to hear the Gospel." Many of the patients, moreover, were visited by "Mr. Lee Won and other missionaries to the Chinese, and thus may have heard the good news of Salvation for the first time while lying on their beds of suffering." The hospital experience furthered the missionary work of the King's Daughters, because "the good seed thus sown, will, we trust, bear . . . *some* fruit to the glory of God our Saviour." The institution was proud that it offered "the double advantages of scientific care and nursing" and the opportunity to "be brought under Christian influences." The evangelical goals of the facility make this and other nineteenth-century hospitals seem more like religious nursing homes than acute-care facilities.[28]

There were a number of interrelated reasons for the long-term nature of most hospital stays. During this period depressions, geographic dislocation, massive immigration, and a short supply of housing created the need to keep patients in the institution for long periods of time. Most patients were drawn from the dependent poor who had few alternatives to the hospital during periods of unemployment. In addition, during the last third of the century, large numbers of immigrants were streaming into the country and settling in isolated religious or ethnic communities that were fairly autonomous and independent of central government control.[29] These communities considered it their responsibility to care for those made dependent by illness, unemployment, or lack of shelter and food, partially because of the immigrants' resistance to what were perceived as alien institutions. "Do not our general hospitals provide for the ill?" it was asked. "It is true they are intended for such purposes, but we often cannot persuade [our countrymen] to enter the institutions."[30]

Although patients in community hospitals were dependent and poor, they were seldom marginal members of the community or outcasts. The patient who was aided in most charity facilities was seen as "worthy" and morally upright. Those in need of care who were defined by lay community workers as morally depraved or of questionable integrity would generally *not* be accepted for care in the community hospital. Those suffering from illnesses like alcoholism or venereal disease – conditions that indicated questionable morality – would be left to the mercies of the city and its prison or public hospital system.[31]

Though patients in the hospital were seen to be in need of moral teachings and reform, they were still stable members of the working class, or "worthy" poor, who might temporarily be in need. Generally they were employed as plumbers, ironworkers, mechanics, domestics, or seamstresses. Those who were permanently unemployed, but considered capable of acquiring a skill or occupation, were generally thought unworthy of hospital admission because of their questionable moral fiber. Patients could not simply admit themselves to the hospital; they needed a sponsor, a prominent community member like a wealthy merchant or minister, who would write a letter to the lay trustee of the hospital attesting to their moral worthiness, and by implication to their stable lower-class position within the community. With the significant exceptions of accident cases, travelers, or visitors to the community who might bypass the scrutiny of the trustees by entering the hospital through the emergency room, the hospital carefully selected those to whom it would extend its charity services.

The importance of community support for small nineteenth-century charity hospitals cannot be stressed enough. In the absence of an organized set of public social services, and in a time before notions of corporate responsibility for health care had developed, the community-supported charity hospitals were an indispensable resource for the community's dependent poor. Granted, most charity hospitals were flawed institutions. As other scholars have pointed out, they were generally underfinanced and understaffed places where cruel treatment and suffering seemed omnipresent. Depending upon the sponsorship and purpose of the hospital, patients were treated with varying combinations of compassion, condescension, and scorn. Often the community's most paternalistic members would organize a hospital with a view toward reforming patients. Treatment sometimes bordered on punishment for working-class patients considered by some trustees to have "underdeveloped or ill-developed character."[32] Because scientifically based medical services were minimal or nonexistent, physicians and surgeons in training quite literally "experimented" or "practiced upon" these patients.

The charity system was also flawed in less obvious ways. Because care often depended upon the goodwill and idiosyncratic decisions of local elites, the system had an extremely haphazard appearance. Some neighborhoods with active churches or wealthy benefactors had an adequate number of hospital services and outpatient dispensaries; other neighborhoods, where the forces of urbanization had destroyed social cohesion, had a severe shortage or absolute absence of health-care services. People could not *expect* to be cared for but could only hope that someone would come to their aid.

Medical care in Brooklyn: the effect of demographic change

By the end of the nineteenth century the system of charity hospitals began to change. Most historians have viewed this change as the result of advances in medical knowledge that attracted more upper-class merchant families to the hospitals for care they could not receive at home. In this book I argue that changes in the hospital were a result as much of changes in the economy and demography as of improved medical knowledge. Furthermore, I argue that, despite improvements in the overall nature of medical care, a certain element of community involvement was lost for laborers and other groups when hospitals changed their focus.

One major change to effect the hospital was the demographic and geographic reorganization of the city. Once composed of a series of relatively independent communities separated by distance and culture, the city became politically and economically integrated as the century progressed, taking the shape we now recognize. Innovations like mass transportation, the telephone, new pavements, and ultimately the automobile began to break down the barriers that had separated distant communities. As a result, communities once composed of residents belonging to a particular ethnic group or sharing a religious belief began to lose some of their wealthier and more socially mobile residents, who took advantage of more attractive housing in newly built and increasingly accessible suburban neighborhoods. Often local practitioners joined with the professionals and other white-collar workers in this move to the suburbs.[33] Those working-class groups who were left behind found themselves without the doctor who had always been around the corner when they or their families needed treatment. In addition, many small neighborhood hospitals, often located on potentially valuable property in downtown areas, were forced to sell their downtown facilities and move to new neighborhoods.

The experience of Brooklyn, New York, illustrates these demographic and geographic changes. Although closely connected to the life of New York City by common economic interests and the newly built

Brooklyn Bridge, Brooklyn was still an independent city in the latter part of the nineteenth century. Known for its profusion of religious institutions and single-family houses, it was often called the "city of churches" or the "city of homes," and portrayed as a civil, bucolic, and sometimes boring alternative to the sinful excesses of Manhattan. The home for many businessmen who commuted to lower Manhattan by bridge or ferry, Brooklyn has been immortalized by the poet Walt Whitman and the evangelical preacher Henry Ward Beecher, both of whom lived there in the mid-century.[34]

Though the elite enclaves of Brooklyn Heights still reflected this bucolic image, by the 1880s most of Brooklyn's communities were composed of poor immigrant working-class neighborhoods spread along the highly industrialized shorelines of the East River and harbor (see Figure 1). Large numbers of Poles, Slovaks, Jews, and Slovenians lived in the Williamsburg and Greenpoint sections of the city; Irish and other Slovaks settled in South Brooklyn; Swedes formed a strong neighborhood just south of Prospect Park; and Syrians created a thriving community on the edge of Brooklyn Heights, near Atlantic Avenue.[35] More separated these neighborhoods than their names: Many communities functioned like independent cities with their own political structure and religious, educational, and health institutions. Their people generally worked in local commercial and industrial enterprises and often had little reason or even ability to leave their neighborhoods

The introduction of the extensive electric and horse-drawn trolley system for which Brooklyn became known, along with other changes in transportation and communication, created the conditions for the city's economic and geographic growth. In fact, by the late nineteenth century, Brooklyn vied with Baltimore and Philadelphia for third place in industrial production behind New York and Chicago. By 1890 Brooklyn could boast major light and heavy manufacturing industries. With a growing population of over 600,000 people, the city employed thousands of workers in needle trades, confectionary and baking production, carpentry, glass, and gas-lamp production. Brooklyn had over 2,500 masons, and more than 3,000 men, women, and children were employed in the Navy Yards. Associated foundries and machine shops employed another 8,000 people in Greenpoint, Williamsburg, and the highly industrial neighborhoods along the shore.[36]

Although the city as a whole prospered economically, many of its laborers barely made a living. Average wages were low, and unemployment was high. An unskilled workman in the light industries could count on only $10 to $12 a week. Were he lucky enough to obtain a skilled laboring position in one of the Navy Yard foundries he might

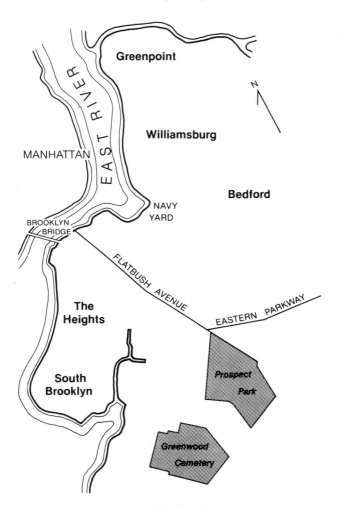

Figure 1. Brooklyn's neighborhoods, ca. 1900.

earn as much as $15 for a sixty-hour week. Women rarely earned
above $7 a week, and children were regularly employed for $4.[37]

In addition, laborers could rarely look forward to many months of
full employment. The degree of unemployment in most manufacturing jobs was staggering. In the New York area in 1900, 13.2 percent of
all workers – male and female – were unemployed for one to three
months. Another 9.3 percent were unemployed for four to six months,
and 2.8 percent more were out of work for seven to twelve months. In

all, 25 percent of the work force could expect to be unemployed in any given year.[38] Because the cost of living for a family of five ranged from $900 to $1,500 a year – or at least $3.10 a day – these wages were far from sufficient.[39] Women sometimes boarded people in their homes in order to earn extra income. But the situation was often so desperate that unemployed and dependent people were regularly thrown onto local charity rolls, or, alternatively, into charity hospitals when illness was added to unemployment. Small community hospitals, organized by local merchants or religious or other civic and moral leaders, were overwhelmed by a needy and increasingly impoverished population.

As the older communities along the coast became crowded with immigrants joining the ranks of the poor and working class, the industrialization and commercialization of the city created a new class of white-collar workers who began to move to large, unpopulated tracts of land farther inland or elsewhere along the coast. From 1880 to 1905, for instance, the population of the city increased by about 125 percent, from just under 600,000 people to over 1.3 million. While arriving immigrants settled in older neighborhoods, white-collar workers moved farther out to East New York, Flatlands, and Bay Ridge, where tracts of land were developed for the first time. East New York and Brownsville experienced a population increase of 42 percent between 1900 and 1905. Similarly, the population of Bay Ridge on the southern rim of the city grew by 50 percent, and the area around Flatbush increased in population by 53 percent in the same period.[40]

These changes did not go unnoticed by members of Brooklyn's health establishment. Lewis Pilcher, a prominent physician in the city, noted that health care was also reacting to the changes around it. "No one can have watched the marvelous events that have been transpiring in our midst . . . without becoming aware of the fact that a new city has arisen and that new social conditions have been created," he remarked.[41] These new conditions created problems as well as possibilities for the health system. As parts of the city became more industrialized many felt that the very physical environment was inappropriate for health facilities. Crowding, noise, and industrial pollution all detracted from the restful image of the hospital. Furthermore, as older communities changed, the nature of the hospital population was bound to alter. An "impending change in the neighborhood from a residential quarter to a business or manufacturing quarter, or to the modifying of the hospital clientele . . . may make a site undesirable for the purpose" of a hospital, noted the authors of one hospital management text of the period.[42]

The arrival of immigrants and the development of the industrial city greatly increased the number of dependent and indigent persons in need of charity and hospital service. Already overcrowded institutions felt tremendous pressure to expand. "With the population and business rapidly increasing in this section of the city," observed one hospital trustee, "the demands made upon our hospital will be proportionately enlarged and . . . the hospital will be taxed to its utmost."[43] As new immigrants arrived, Norwegian, Jewish, Lutheran, German, and other community leaders planned for the creation of new services.

The expansion in manufacturing also caused a large increase in work-related injuries. Hospitals and dispensaries located close to an industrial hub like Greenpoint, and serving primarily working-class patients, found their emergency rooms crowded with people who had been hit by trolleys or injured while working in factories or doing construction jobs.[44] In 1891 the ambulance of the Methodist Hospital brought in nearly a thousand laborers from the surrounding area of the city, where there was a great deal of construction going on. Methodist's 1891 *Annual Report* stated that "those termed 'laborers' were the most numerous class [of patients]. They were largely 'accident cases' brought in by our ambulance."[45] In 1892, 39 percent of Brooklyn Hospital's patients were brought in by ambulance. By 1911 the ambulance still brought in one of every five patients.

By 1905 Brooklyn comprised 120 square miles running 12 miles from east to west and 10 miles from north to south. An injured or sick worker was often far from the hospitals located in the older sections of the city. Only eighteen horse-drawn ambulances serviced Brooklyn, and they were extremely haphazard and slow. A study of the city's ambulance facilities noted that the ambulance of the Norwegian Hospital "often runs 10 to 12 miles in going and returning with a patient." Given the poor conditions of many unpaved and muddy streets, it was not unusual for some ambulance "runs" to last six to eight hours.[46]

Although the old hospitals and ambulance services were inadequate, new suburban neighborhoods had no hospitals at all to provide emergency care for those moving there and the working class who served them. Hospitals were generally located along the coast in older working-class communities. An important study done in 1908 noted that "a line two miles long drawn in a circle . . . reaches 15 out of the city's general hospitals . . . and within a two and a half mile radius every hospital except two will be included."[47] It was clear that new hospitals needed to be built if emergency and ambulance services were to be provided to persons living and working in the outlying suburban areas.

Shifts in the *social* organization of the city also affected health care. As we have seen, the old nineteenth-century walking city was beginning to give way to the present-day industrial city. The downtown area of Brooklyn, previously a sleepy district serving the wealthy residents of Brooklyn Heights, was becoming the hub of a bustling and crowded shopping district. The construction of the Brooklyn Bridge in the 1880s, the development of an extensive electric trolley system, and the introduction of elevated railroad lines brought thousands of Brooklynites to this downtown shopping area. Brooklyn ceased to be a conglomeration of independent neighborhoods and began to take on many of the aspects of a modern city with an integrated economic and social life. Major construction destroyed residences of all kinds. The working class, unable to afford new suburban housing, was forced into more crowded slums, whereas white-collar workers were able to move farther out to Prospect Park and beyond. Planners noted that "the demands of business and trade are constantly encroaching upon the fringes of the residential sections." In the decade between 1880 and 1890, when the population of Brooklyn was increasing by 50 percent, the population of two wards in the downtown neighborhoods actually decreased. Between 1890 and 1900 the population of four more adjacent downtown wards decreased as workers widened streets for increased traffic, converted buildings for commercial use, and rebuilt large areas to accommodate department stores and municipal offices.[48] "Every year sees old houses here turned into stores or factories, or torn down to make way for business blocks," one observer noted. The owners of major department stores, such as Abraham and Straus, bought up acres of land in the neighborhood to construct stores, storage buildings, and shipping depots.[49] Rental costs for scarcer apartments and space soared, further forcing the middle class out and pushing the growing number of poor immigrants into fewer and fewer overcrowded buildings.

Health institutions were affected by these changes in a variety of ways. The Brooklyn Eye and Ear Hospital was directly involved when Livingston Street, soon to become a major thoroughfare, was widened in 1905. "By the widening of Livingston Street," the hospital's *Annual Report* noted in 1906, "the hospital was deprived of thirty feet of frontage." To avoid having to move, the hospital was forced to buy expensive additional space on Schermerhorn Street.[50] Some institutions did move to new locations. The leadership of the Kings County Medical Society, the official society of Brooklyn's physicians, decided that its old headquarters near the now bustling Brooklyn Bridge was too small and noisy for the society's growing membership. In 1894–1895, the membership was asked to choose between a location in the hub of the downtown area near Fulton Street and Flatbush Avenue and "a site further uptown" in the newly opened Bedford region. "This very important question eventually settled itself," reported William Browning, an important figure in the society. "No satisfactory location near [downtown] was found at any figure within our means."[51] Members decided that "the opening up of the Nassau trolley system and the connection of the Brighton Beach steam road with the Kings County Elevator gave a good choice of sites in the Bedford region." The major advantage of the newer neighborhood was that it was "central, accessible and not too expensive."[52]

The increasing cost of downtown land and the physical deterioration of growing commercial and industrial neighborhoods forced some facilities into a state of perpetual motion. The Memorial Hospital for Women and Children moved no fewer than six times in a period of eight years. First located in the "factory district" near Myrtle Avenue and Grand Street, this facility began a migration that finally ended in the then fashionable and newer Bedford neighborhood.[53] The Bushwick and East Brooklyn Dispensary was also forced to "buy a plot elsewhere that will be . . . less expensive."[54]

Institutions were forced to move not only because land became scarce and expensive: Some found that the social and moral character of the central city was unsuitable for their charity facilities. "We are perforce obliged to relinquish our present situation," reported the secretary of one women's hospital. "The proximity of Washington Street, which is so crowded a thoroughfare, the passage of seven lines of cars before our doors . . . the near presence of saloons which induce . . . hangers-on and purposeless lounging on street corners makes our building very undesirable for our uses."[55]

Almost universally, institutions were relocated from the older neighborhoods near the shoreline to the developing areas farther inland. This generally meant that institutions were moving away from working-class areas into middle-class and white-collar neighborhoods. As the city expanded, white-collar workers moved into the heart of Kings County, toward farms and villages near Crown Heights, Flatbush, Flatlands, and Canarsie, and into the areas north and south of Eastern Parkway. A number of small health institutions moved to this area as well. Land was relatively cheap, transportation was available, and the area, with its tree-lined streets and three-story brownstone and white-stone buildings, was commodious. The neighborhood boasted such amenities as Prospect Park, Eastern Parkway, and the Brooklyn Academy of Music.[56] "We look to the new wards, in the neighborhood of . . . Park Place and Classon Avenue . . . with longing eyes," said the president of Brooklyn's Women's Homeopathic Hospital.[57]

Rather than welcoming changes in the city, private community doctors often found the physical reorganization of the city threatening to their practices. In 1910 a group of doctors protested the planned destruction of their homes and offices in the downtown section of the city. Two blocks on Schermerhorn Street were to be razed in order to make room for a new courthouse and plaza. The thirty physicians who practiced there protested to the Kings County Medical Society that not only would their homes be destroyed by the demolition, but their very livelihoods would be threatened as well. They requested that the society pass a resolution against the demolition.

The basis for the physicians' protest was that a doctor's "work differs from any other calling" in that his "daily bread depends upon his professional acquaintances" and local patients. "If a doctor abandons his location," argued the practitioners, "it is impossible to notify all his patients of his new address." Otherwise loyal patients might quickly abandon a physician who was forced to move too far away, and this would seriously undermine the doctor's ability to earn a living. Patients "remember a doctor's location and return to consult him even though they may not remember his name," the petitioners pointed out. If the physicians left the area, the practices that had taken them so long to build up might easily be lost.[58]

The most pressing problem for the doctors was the lack of available land in the immediate area upon which to establish new offices and homes. The "topography of Brooklyn," they complained, "makes it impossible . . . to find new locations within a radius of a few blocks of [our] present offices." Downtown land was already divided to such an extent that there was simply no room. After Schermerhorn Street was destroyed, they observed, "there remains in the vicinity only property which is already occupied by doctors, the business property of Montague, Remsen and Court Streets, or the very large and expensive property of the Heights, which are beyond the reach of a doctor's income, either in rental or purchase price." Also, "on the other side . . . are stables, factories, and poor dwellings," which were not only inappropriate for the doctors' offices but also totally inaccessible to paying clientele.[59]

The Medical Society, which had left the area a decade earlier, quickly passed the resolution condemning the construction of the court house. But it had little effect on the builders who were reorganizing the downtown. Along with other physicians, the doctors on Schermerhorn Street moved away to the newly developing suburban areas.

A number of technological changes facilitated the doctors' departure from the center city. The widespread introduction of the telephone allowed suburban doctors to maintain their ties with their patients and colleagues in the older neighborhood. Whereas less than 3 percent of the city's physicians had telephone services in 1890, 97 percent of doctors had telephones by 1918. Because of the trolley some doctors were able for the first time to move to the suburbs and still maintain contact with older clients downtown. Those doctors unable to maintain both a house and an office in the downtown area sometimes rented office space downtown and commuted to work each morning along with thousands of other white-collar workers.[60] Other doctors, who chose to establish a new practice among families more affluent than those they had served in the older walking city, moved to the Bedford and Crown Heights area. In 1890, before the introduction of the electric trolley, such suburban streets as Eastern Parkway, Halsey Avenue, and Hancock Street had fewer than five physicians living on them; by 1918 all of these avenues had more than forty doctors each (see Table 1). In 1890 the streets listed in Table 1 housed only 16.7 percent of the offices of physicians of Brooklyn; by 1918 these same streets housed 29 percent of the city's doctors.[61]

Despite the promise of continued accessibility between doctors and patients, when doctors moved away, doctors' services actually became less accessible to the majority of the city's poor. A mammoth health survey of New York and Brooklyn conducted in 1890 by the Census Office contained statistics that documented what had long been apparent to many – that the older, poorer neighborhoods lining the East River and harbor, from Greenpoint to Redhook, were afflicted with the severest of health problems. Crowded living conditions, poor housing, lack of heat, polluted water, and inadequate sanitation took their toll on the health and lives of the working-class populations in these areas. John S. Billings and the Census Office showed in a detailed, ward-by-ward survey that pneumonia, diphtheria, croup, scarlet fever, measles, whooping cough, and malarial fever were major killers of people living in the industrial and port facilities along the water's edge. With the exception of the wealthy area around the Heights, the shoreline of the city had death and sickness rates well above the city's average.[62] Whereas the city as a whole had a death rate of just under 25 per 1,000 for the period 1884 to 1890, some wards in Greenpoint had death rates twice as high. A section of Ward 17 encompassing the northernmost portion of heavily industrialized Greenpoint had a death rate that exceeded 50 per 1,000. Most areas in South Brooklyn, a region of swamps, shacks, and port facilities, had death rates of over 30

Table 1. *Number of physicians with offices on selected streets in the new wards for 1890, 1900, 1910, and 1918*

Street	1890	1900	1910	1918
Bedford Avenue	28	33	39	44
Bergen Street	4	15	29	23
Bushwick Avenue	9	29	45	56
Clinton Street	39	57	64	48
Dean Street	3	10	19	28
Eastern Parkway	—	—	10	47
Gates Avenue	9	20	18	22
Greene Avenue	22	23	49	48
Halsey Avenue	4	26	48	42
Hancock Street	4	23	41	48
Jefferson Avenue	5	20	26	28
Lafayette Avenue	16	21	26	28
McDonough Street	4	20	22	33
Ninth Street	10	23	26	27
Park Place	1	5	15	30
Putnam Avenue	4	12	15	21
St. John's Place	3	5	11	24
St. Mark's Avenue	5	12	34	37
Schermerhorn Street	17	24	23	22
Stone Avenue	—	4	18	26
Union Street	10	26	33	28
Washington Avenue	9	15	28	22

Notes: Streets with 20 or more physicians practicing on them in 1918 were selected from the lists of Brooklyn physicians. A dash indicates no data.
Source: "Street Lists of Brooklyn Physicians," *Medical Directories,* 1890, 1900, 1910, 1918.

per 1,000 and disease rates significantly higher than those of the inland portions of the city (see Figure 2).[63]

Although morbidity and mortality rates were exceedingly high in older neighborhoods, they were very low in the newer areas to which doctors were moving. In some sections death rates were as low as 16 per 1,000, and nearly all the newer neighborhoods experienced rates well below the city average.[64]

The migration of private physicians to the newly opened areas affected health services in a very significant way. Poorer neighborhoods, never well supplied with private practitioners, experienced a further decrease in services. One small area near the Navy Yard, for instance, was generally noted as one of the city's poorest and least healthy.[65] This area of 21,000 people, mostly Irish workers and their families, had

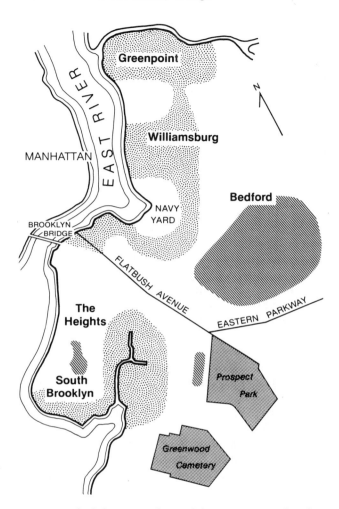

Figure 2. Areas to which large numbers of doctors migrated and areas with high mortality rates. Lines indicate doctors' new neighborhoods and dots indicate working-class and high-mortality neighborhoods.

only thirteen physicians' offices in 1890. By 1918 only five elderly physicians still practiced there.[66] Other poor areas of the city experienced a similar decrease in physicians' offices. Although the number of doctors more than doubled in the city during the period 1890–1918, older, poorer, and more medically needy areas found themselves with fewer physicians.[67]

The transformation of the city from a series of small communities relatively isolated from each other to a major industrial center connected by a mass-transportation system, telephones, paved roads, and, ultimately, automobiles had a serious impact on health services. The development of socioeconomically distinct neighborhoods of inner-city poor and wealthier "suburbanites" destroyed the community-practice model of health care. Doctors, previously associated with geographically defined walking neighborhoods, were pressed by the forces of urban growth to move with other white-collar workers away from the center of the city to the newer suburban areas. Working-class neighborhoods were abandoned for areas like "Pill Hill" or "Doctor's Row" in the Crown Heights area of Brooklyn. Our modern designation of entire regions of Brooklyn and other cities as "medically underserved areas" underscores the tragic consequences of this ongoing suburbanization process.

The removal of the physician from the neighborhood had a subtler impact on the quality of care. The intimate relationship between the practitioner and the community that characterized nineteenth-century practice began to break down. Because the nineteenth-century doctor had lived in the community where he practiced, he was engaged in its church, school, and political life. His involvement in the life of the community strengthened the bonds of trust between him and his patients. As the new industrial and commercial city gave rise to socioeconomically segregated neighborhoods, people could no longer beckon the doctor from around the corner to preside at the family's births and deaths. The relationship between patient and physician was soon to become more professional and distant. The doctor became an outsider whose authority was based upon his scientific expertise, not upon his status as a trusted member of the community. Though patients gained much from his increased scientific knowledge, they stood to lose a great deal as a result of the doctor's physical and emotional distance from them.

Demographic changes brought physical distance between patients and hospitals as well. Some institutions moved to new communities far from the working class, where they developed services appropriate to the needs of the middle class but often lacked the emergency and other services needed by working-class people employed in the area. The hospitals that remained in the working-class neighborhoods changed as well. Their wealthy merchant-trustees, some of whom also left the neighborhood, easily lost touch with the needs of the communities their hospitals served. Away from their communities, these trustees were more easily swayed by economic and political pressures that often ran counter to the needs of their hospitals' patients.

The processes that would alter the character of health-care delivery in the city had begun. Brooklyn had changed from a rural town to a major industrial and merchant center. In 1898 Brooklyn would merge with New York across the East River and become part of the country's preeminent city. In the process the health system would become even more alienating and less connected to communities than it had been.

The changes outlined in this chapter were the result of economic and demographic forces generally outside the control of the people involved. The health institutions that were affected responded as they had to if they were to survive. Some moved. Some disappeared. As will be discussed elsewhere, some made changes in services and pay arrangements in order to survive.

But other social forces also created major problems for doctors, trustees, and workers in the health system. Perhaps the most dramatic event to affect hospitals was the severe economic depression that occurred between 1893 and 1897. This national crisis affected the financial structure and organization of many small charity systems in ways that we can still observe today. The next chapter illustrates the profound effect of a rapidly changing general economy on small charity hospitals.

2   Embattled benefactors:
the crisis in hospital financing

The 1890s were hardly gay for the majority of Americans. Before the decade was halfway completed an economic depression of unheard-of magnitude had swept the country and threatened the very existence of millions of blue-collar workers, small businessmen, and even bankers. Following the panic of 1893, over 600 banks closed, 16,000 business firms went bankrupt, and 2.5 million laborers were suddenly jobless. The 1,300 strikes by workers in most heavy industries, coupled with the obvious plight of thousands of workers who marched on Washington in "General" Coxey's army, led one senator to fear that the country was "on the verge of revolution."[1]

In New York, the effect of the Depression was extremely severe. "Times were hard," recalled Lillian Wald, the famous founder of the Henry Street Settlement. "In the summer the miseries due to unemployment and rising rents and prices began to be apparent, but the pinch came with the cold weather." The winter of 1893–1894, the first of a depression that was to last through 1897, was most memorable to Wald. She observed firsthand "the extraordinary sufferings and the variety of pain and poverty" of those living in the tenements of New York's lower East Side.[2]

The city's merchants were also severely affected by the Depression, as were the small charity institutions that depended upon their contributions. Coming on the heels of a steady rise in the costs of supplies, fuel, and food, the shock of reduced support was disruptive and, for some facilities, fatal. The tenuous hospital-financing system depended upon philanthropy, and its susceptibility to economic downturns was clearly illustrated during the Depression years. A long-term effort among trustees, administrators, and others involved in charity to reform the financial base of health facilities commenced in the wake of the Depression.

Hospital financing at the turn of the century

Before the 1890s Depression, charity hospitals traditionally depended upon a number of diverse sources for their financial support (see Table 2).

April, 1917
Vol. III, No. 3

HOSPITAL MANAGEMENT

608 S. Dearborn
Street,
Chicago

Published in the Interest of Executives in Every Department of Hospital Work

This Young Fellow Has Been Growing Right Out of His Clothes

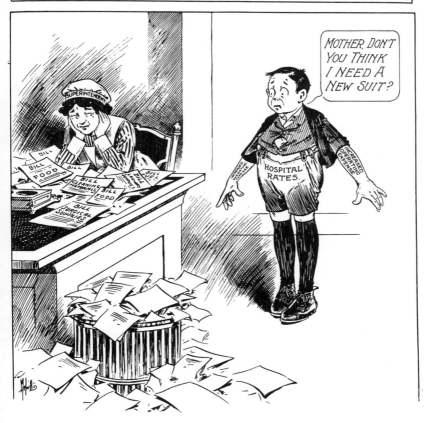

Growing costs were a persistent problem for hospital administrators during the Progressive era. Here the cartoonist shows a worried administrator facing the prospect of increasing her hospital's charges to patients. Before the 1920s, a very large proportion of head administrators were women.

Table 2. *Sources of income for selected hospitals, 1889 and 1890*

Hospital	Dividends & invested programs		Donations		Legacies		Hosp. Sat. & Sun Assoc.[a]	
	1889	1890	1889	1890	1889	1890	1889	1890
Mass. General Hospital								
$	110,155	84,793	11,850	13,496	0	0	0	0
% of budget	75	66	8	11	0	0	0	0
St. Luke's Hospital								
$	31,899	34,795	12,419	100,876	4,285	136,580	7,789	8,671
% of budget	29	11	11	33	4	45	7	3
Presbyterian Hosp., N.Y.								
$	44,996	34,622	73,404	235,034	2,500	235	0	0
% of budget	35	12	57	84	2	0	0	0
University of Penn.								
$	28,320	27,843	2,225	29,748	0	5,000	0	0
% of budget	49	33	4	35	0	6	0	0
Rhode Island Hospital								
$	26,512	27,455	3,143	5,903	2,000	250	1,307	1,408
% of budget	63	63	7	13	5	1	3	3

Harper Hosp., Detroit								
$	3,100	7,952	1,676	859	0	0	0	0
% of budget	11	21	6	2	0	0	0	0
Maine General Hospital								
$	8,491	8,379	5,948	3,782	1,250	4,600	783	983
% of budget	22	22	15	10	3	12	2	3
Methodist Hosp., Brooklyn								
$	3,274	4,357	35,744	22,404	0	0	0	0
% of budget	6	10	66	51	0	0	0	0
City Hospital, Worcester								
$	9,465	10,480	0	0	0	0	0	0
% of budget	30	32	0	0	0	0	0	0
Cambridge Hosp., Mass.								
$	2,860	4,189	17,059	14,958	20,000	0	0	0
% of budget	7	15	39	55	46	0	0	0

Table 2. (continued)

Hospital	Patients' payments		Misc. receipts[b]		Totals		Investment & endowment	
	1889	1890	1889	1890	1889	1890	1889	1890
Mass. General Hospital								
$	24,824	29,438	0	0	146,829	127,727	1,874,811	1,933,502
% of budget	16	23	0	0	99[c]	100		
St. Luke's Hospital								
$	19,657	25,264	34,788	390	110,839	306,577	659,089	835,670
% of budget	18	8	31	0	100	100		
Presbyterian Hosp., N.Y.								
$	8,192	6,458	0	4,676	129,094	281,027	0	0
% of budget	6	2	0	2	100	100		
University of Penn.								
$	21,336	21,006	5,937	919	57,818	84,517	0	0
% of budget	37	25	10	1	100	100		
Rhode Island Hospital								
$	8,674	8,383	550	466	42,187	43,867	451,245	452,845
% of budget	20	19	1	1	99	100		

Harper Hosp., Detroit								
$	21,625	27,674	1,044	779	27,445	37,263	50,000	133,500
% of budget	79[d]	74[d]	4	2	100	99	0	0
Maine General Hospital								
$	17,703	15,410	5,241	5,294	39,417	38,448	0	0
% of budget	45	40	13	14	100	101		
Methodist Hosp., Brooklyn								
$	0	5,721	15,479	11,712	54,497	44,195	100,000	113,723
% of budget	0	13	28	27	100	101		
City Hospital, Worcester								
$	4,002	4,775	17,805	17,755	31,271	33,011	226,832	227,962
% of budget	13	14	57	54	100	100		
Cambridge Hosp., Mass.								
$	3,205	3,266	632	4,764	43,756	27,177	95,232	104,622
% of budget	7	12	1	18	100	100		

[a] The Hospital Saturday and Sunday Association was a charitable organization that collected funds for member institutions on the Sabbath – Saturday or Sunday. It antedated the United Hospital Fund.
[b] For Worcester, St. Luke's, Pennsylvania, Cambridge and Methodist hospitals, this category was partly made up of public funds donated by the city. For the other institutions, the meaning of the column is unclear.
[c] Because of rounding, percentages do not always total to 100.
[d] Because Harper Hospital was a private institution, receipts from its patients constituted an unusually large percentage of its income.

Source: Henry C. Burdett, *Hospitals and Asylums of the World,* vol. 3 (London: J. & A. Churchill, 1893), pp. 718–791.

First, there were the private sources – philanthropic giving, endowments, and investments in property – which accounted for the vast bulk of the institutions' income. A few large established facilities like the Massachusetts General Hospital derived as much as 75 percent of their income from dividends on property alone; other institutions gathered most of their income from a combination of investments, legacies, donations, and miscellaneous patient payments. Contributions from private philanthropists, along with patient payments, generally covered the daily costs of food, fuel, salaries, construction, and medical supplies. In addition, in New York and Brooklyn and other localities, municipal and state departments of public charities reimbursed hospitals for the care of the city's indigent. In the middle years of the nineteenth century, when the costs for maintenance and medical care remained relatively small, these sources of income were sufficient. Small deficits left at the end of the year were usually covered by donations derived from benefits and appeals or from willing trustees, who saw themselves as stewards for the poor.

For a long time, these deficits were not viewed with alarm but were seen as responsible for the financial solvency of many nineteenth-century charity facilities: They lent legitimacy to appeals for donations and construction drives by providing evidence that more money was required for the needy. Had these institutions been solvent, they could hardly have asked for financial help. Modest and temporary poverty was as much a characteristic of nineteenth-century hospitals as it was a characteristic of the people hospitals sought to serve. As one trustee observed, the "deficit and consequent debt [of the hospital represented] the most marked evidence of the spirit that has inspired its management."[3] Very often ladies' auxiliaries sponsored dances, lectures, and teas to make up the deficits of their favorite institutions. Churches took up special "Saturday and Sunday" collections, and hospitals often used their end-of-the-year financial reports to motivate the benevolent to give money in the spirit of Christmas.

Often the bid for contributions to make up the deficit included a plea for funds to construct new facilities or to expand in order to meet the increased demands posed by immigration. Although the Methodist Hospital in Brooklyn had the largest endowment fund of any Brooklyn hospital, its 1890 *Annual Report* stated that even more money was needed to open new portions of the hospital. Fund raising became an increasingly large task for hospital administrators. The hospital "being without adequate endowment," Methodist's superintendent noted, he had to "add to his duties those of a financial agent, and incur the expense of travelling widely in the interest of the institution."[4] Generally the call for funds was pitched to appeal to the humanitarian spirit in people. In 1889 Brooklyn Throat Hospital's *Annual Report* stated that "the beneficent work of the Hospital is growing larger day by day [and] it is [the trustees'] right to ask the cooperative support of . . . philanthropic men and women."[5] Thomas Kenna, president of the Long Island Throat and Lung Hospital, repeated a similar theme: "Let us hope that the charitable and humane among our citizens, realizing the broad scope of our operations and the benevolent character of our work, may assist in making a new hospital structure built . . . in the near future."[6]

Because no amount of fund raising could make up the deficits created by growing costs in the 1890s, many administrators and trustees were forced to face the possibility of insolvency. Deficits, long considered a necessary inconvenience, became defined as a major problem for the first time.[7] Throughout the city, hospital administrators began to complain more strenuously of deficits, inability to meet bills, and the evaporation of contributions. They often cited the Depression as the cause. In a desperate appeal for funds in 1899, the superintendent of the Memorial Hospital for Women and Children remembered that when the "financial depression struck this land, we were obliged to struggle on as best we could."[8] "Our hospital, in common with all other [such] Institutions, has felt this year more particularly the financial depression," remarked the authors of the Memorial Hospital's *Annual Report* as late as 1898.[9]

Before the 1890s the cost of running a community charity hospital was still relatively low, and a few wealthy benefactors were sufficient to guarantee the financial stability of an institution. Some of the smaller specialty and general hospitals ran for less than $3,000 per year. In 1889, for instance, the Brooklyn Throat Hospital provided limited inpatient and extensive outpatient services for over 23,000 patients while spending only $2,906. Institutions that provided longer-term care, such as Memorial Hospital for Women and Homeopathic Maternity Hospital, began the 1890s with a budget of less than $83,000 each for the care of the expectant mothers in their 100-bed hospitals. Even the largest of Brooklyn's hospitals had relatively small budgets in the early nineties. Brooklyn Hospital, for instance, expended less than $40,000 for its 100-bed facility in 1892 (see Table 3); the new Methodist Hospital's disbursements were only $44,000 in the 1890 fiscal year.

In Manhattan the situation was similar. Though there were a number of large institutions such as Mount Sinai, St. Luke's, Roosevelt, and New York Hospital, where the total expenses exceeded $100,000 per year, most hospitals ran for considerably less. One 1896 survey of thirty-five hospitals in Manhattan revealed that twenty-two had total yearly expenditures of less than $30,000 and only thirteen spent more

Table 3. *Some statistics for the Brooklyn Hospital for the years 1885 to 1915*

Year	Average patient stay (days)	Expenses ($)	Number of patients	Average cost per day ($)	Number of days' treatment
1885	31.7	20,239	820	0.78	25,978
1890	29.6	29,796	1,131	0.89	33,431
1895	29.4	44,022	1,240	1.21	36,429
1900	20.1	66,361	2,279	1.42	45,796
1905	20.7	74,538	2,174	1.65	45,117
1910	17.7	86,950	2,574	1.90	45,552
1915	15.6	123,385	2,844	2.78	44,316

Source: Brooklyn Hospital, *Annual Reports*, 1910, 1915, p. 12.

Table 4. *Total expenditures of thirty-five Manhattan hospitals for the year ending September 30, 1896*

Expenditures (in thousands of dollars)	Number of hospitals
0–10	4
11–20	7
21–30	11
31–40	2
41–50	2
51–60	0
61–70	2
71–80	1
81–90	1
91–100	2
101+	3

Source: Statement of Expenditures, Resources and Work of the Hospitals Connected with the Saturday and Sunday Association of New York City, 1896, in New York Hospital Archives, Papers, 1897, folder: 1897, fiscal–finance committee.

than that. Of the thirty-five hospitals surveyed, the median expenditure was just below $28,000 and the mean was $35,000 per year (see Table 4).

During the Progressive era the expenditures necessary for maintaining institutions skyrocketed. Between 1890 and 1899, for instance, Memorial Hospital increased its expenditures nearly 400 percent as costs grew from just over $7,200 to over $27,000; Homeopathic Maternity saw its expenditures grow from $8,300 in 1889 to over $14,000 by 1899. Expenditures at the Eye and Ear grew fivefold from $10,000 in 1896 to over $55,000 by 1913. Likewise, Methodist's expenditures nearly doubled during the 1890s, and Brooklyn Hospital's costs quadrupled between 1892 and 1915.

A number of factors explain this rapid inflationary spiral. First of all, the Depression brought into focus the long-term rise in the costs of medical supplies. Some administrators saw the "increased costs of supplies and materials made necessary by advancing science" as the most significant factor affecting hospital costs.[10] At Methodist Hospital, for instance, the superintendent observed in 1894 that many "first class surgical instruments have been placed in our cabinets, which now contain several thousand dollars worth."[11]

A brief inspection of the expenditures of Brooklyn Hospital indicates the complex nature of cost inflation during this period. At Brooklyn Hospital, no particular item was solely responsible for the increasing costs. The proportions of the whole budget expended for payroll, food, fuel, furnishings, repairs, training school, ambulance support, and miscellaneous costs show surprising consistency. The only expense that showed significant change during the period was the category "medical supplies." This expense grew from just over 7 percent of the budget in 1892 to 15 percent by 1900; after the turn of the century, however, the amount of the hospital's budget devoted to this category stabilized at between 9 and 12 percent. After an initial period of investment in equipment, then, it appears that Brooklyn Hospital did not incur a continually spiraling rise in the percentage of its budget devoted to supplies. Given the rapidly rising outlays for all expenses and the relative stability of proportions devoted to particular categories of expenditure, rising costs were not the only problem.

For many hospitals the increased demand for services caused by the Depression really made costs skyrocket. "The poor we have always with us and the greater the necessity for relief, the greater will the demand be upon all charitable institutions for that relief," declared the secretary of Brooklyn Maternity in 1896. "The public heart is more open to sympathy . . . than ever before, and so it is that the demand is becoming greater each year upon us."[12]

The Depression had indeed created greater need, and thousands of indigent and working-class persons flocked to hospitals for direct aid and support. Institutions noted record growths in their patient populations during the 1890s. "The greatest annual increase," observed the *Annual Report* of the Eye and Ear, "was in 1894."[13] The Nursery and Infants' Hospital noted a similar trend. "In reviewing the records of the past twelve months [of 1895], we find that . . . we have had many more applications for admission of children than we could possibly accommodate," commented this institution's president. "The times have been hard. We have done what we could, at times we have been much overcrowded, but it is hard to turn away from any appeals for aid, and only from lack of room and funds . . . we have done so."[14]

The specialty and special-purpose hospitals felt the most immediate effects of the Depression. Its problems were particularly acute for women and children, among the most poorly paid and dependent of the city's population: The Memorial Hospital for Women and Children nearly quadrupled its patient loads between 1892 and 1898, and the number of patients treated at Nursery and Infants' Hospital doubled between 1892 and 1895.

Another reason for the financial crisis was the absolute and relative decline in the amount of income gathered from the city's hard-pressed philanthropists. Central Throat Hospital and the Brooklyn Maternity, for instance, experienced serious decreases in donations during the Depression years of the 1890s. At the tiny Central Throat Hospital donations dropped from 55 percent of the annual income in 1893 to almost nothing in 1894. Similarly, Brooklyn Maternity saw the percentage of its income derived from various philanthropies drop precipitously between 1894 and 1895. Even the city's oldest and most prestigious institutions suffered as the Depression progressed. "The past year has been without legacy or gift," noted the director of the Brooklyn Eye and Ear Hospital in 1898.[15] William Low, president of the Brooklyn Hospital, complained in the 1895 *Annual Report*: "On the financial side, we have not been able to meet our expenses."[16] (See Figures 3, 4, and 5 for examples of the changing importance of charitable donations during the Progressive era.)

Those hospitals which had to go into debt to meet their expenses were faced with the added problem of huge interest payments. By 1902 the editors of a major nursing journal pointed out that "the [Brooklyn] hospital [had] to pay nearly $2,000 a year interest on its loans."[17] But Brooklyn Hospital's interest payments were trivial in comparison to those of some of the larger institutions. New York Hospital's floating debt of $650,000 was costing the board of governors $26,000 a year in interest charges alone, equal to the entire yearly budget of most Manhattan hospitals.[18]

Other health-care institutions besides hospitals experienced serious declines in income as a result of a drop in contributions. The Board of Managers of the Brooklyn Central Dispensary stated: "It has been customary to call the attention of the generous . . . to our work. Few have come to our assistance."[19] The managers of the Brooklyn Eye and Ear Hospital described the paradox that plagued many hospitals during the depression years: "Not only are the demands upon the Hospital greater and expenses constantly increasing, but the sources of revenue from individual subscriptions are diminishing . . . Of the ninety subscribers to the buying and fitting up of the Hospital in 1882 . . . fully one-half have died; only two of this number left bequests to the Hospital."[20]

At the very time when hospital trustees were reeling from the rapidly rising costs of hospital care, the growth in patient loads spurred some facilities to engage in unwise efforts to expand their services. Construction drives, seemingly contraindicated by a chronic financial crisis, were initiated at a number of facilities. It was felt that in hard

Difference in thousands of dollars

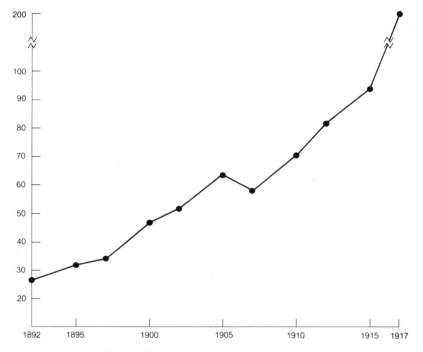

Figure 3. Net difference between income derived from charity and total income, in thousands of dollars, for Brooklyn Hospital, 1892–1917. (*Source*: Brooklyn Hospital, *Annual Reports*, 1892–1917.)

times contributors were more likely to donate buildings, wings, and wards that might bear their names than to contribute to the general fund for hospital maintenance and services. Sometimes expansion was undertaken even at the expense of the institution's long-term solvency: "The contemplated improvements and enlargement of the Hospital," it was observed at the Eye and Ear Hospital, "will necessitate using part of the invested fund, unless contributions are especially made to meet the outlay."[21] At the Brooklyn Hospital, "the work of renovating the Hospital buildings and renewing the equipment has been actively continued . . . the expense of which has been wholly defrayed by members of the Board of Trustees."[22] In 1902 the board of governors at New York Hospital noted that their extraordinary debt was created in part by the erection of a "new Hospital and Administration Building, which [was] still incomplete."[23]

% of total income

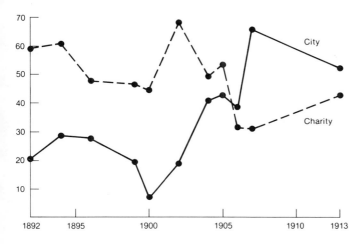

Figure 4. Sources of income for Brooklyn Nursery and Infants' Hospital, 1892–1913, in percentages of total income. (*Source:* Brooklyn Nursery and Infants' Hospital, *Annual Reports*, 1892–1913.)

Expanding at the very time when costs were rising so rapidly was like pouring gasoline on a small fire. It further accelerated a growing crisis in hospital finance. With "these magnificent new hospital buildings," noted a perceptive observer, "has come an increased cost . . . that is little short of appalling."[24] But hospitals often engaged in this appalling activity even in the face of recognized danger. "The difficulty of meeting our daily disbursements was so great that many thought it unwise to attempt anything more," remarked the superintendent of Methodist Hospital in 1894. But "Mr. George Barlow's gift of $1,000 led them to think otherwise," and a drive to secure new building funds was begun.[25]

By the early 1900s, the annual deficits incurred by most hospitals in New York City became a generally recognized problem among the city's hospital trustees, administrators, and even charity workers. A series of articles by Frank Tucker in the journal *Charities* in 1904 prompted a serious discussion of this issue. The Association for Improving the Condition of the Poor recognized the widespread concern over deficits and sponsored, on March 23, 1905, a "Conference on Hospital Needs and Hospital Finances." In the announcement for the meeting, the conference sponsors noted that "heavy annual deficits are

% of total income

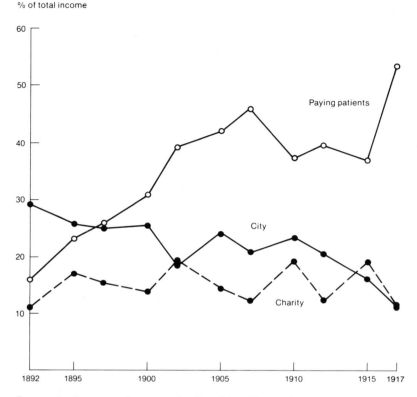

Figure 5. Sources of income for Brooklyn Hospital, 1892–1917, in percentages of total income. (*Source*: Brooklyn Hospital, *Annual Reports*, 1892–1917.)

the rule rather than the exception [for the hospitals of New York City]."[26] Other observers pointed out that "the financial problem of the private hospitals of New York grows as it is studied."[27]

The new trustees

To many trustees, the crisis in hospital finance that developed during the Progressive era simply indicated the need to gather larger donations. Trustees were not used to thinking primarily about money and were often reluctant to look at the unsteady financial base upon which hospitals rested. When faced with the hospitals' need for money, they thought in terms of the kind of personalized financing that had proven successful for so long. In 1893 at Brooklyn Hospital, for instance, the treasurer promptly responded to the growing deficit by expanding the subscription list. William Low, president of the trustees, announced that "names of persons are desired who are willing to aid in guaranteeing payment of any deficiency that may occur during the current year." This group of patrons, Low noted, was to "contribute equally, and no one [would] be called upon for more than one hundred dollars."[28]

By the 1890s even the most prestigious institutions recognized that the resources of the wealthy merchants upon whom they depended were strained and that charity had to be sought from different or less affluent members of society. This perception led to an increase in the kind of minor fund-raising activities that had generally occurred at the end of the year. At Brooklyn Maternity Hospital, a series of talks, fairs, parlor meetings, readings, and cake sales were presented to collect some revenue. A cake sale at Mrs. Sidney Sternbuck's house netted $69 for the hard-pressed institution, and Mr. Silas Pratt's reading of the allegory "America" produced nearly $200. For the Maternity, Mrs. Plummer's "Familiar Talk on Egypt and Palestine" gathered in $80; the Parlor Fair at Mrs. W. B. Pierson's house collected another $52.[29] Although these benefits and drives were hardly new, they were pursued with an urgency that illustrated the deepening financial crisis affecting the city's hospitals.[30]

It became clear to many that the simple goodwill that characterized benefits and bake sales could not avert the crisis. Many thought that by expanding the size of the board of trustees they could continue the kind of funding through philanthropy that had previously characterized hospital finance. Whereas trustees were selected in the past for their commitment to the institution and to charity care, new trustees were selected primarily for their money. A larger number of trustees ensured a larger pool of potential contributors, both from the new trustees themselves and from the new networks of wealthy people that the hospital could approach through them. The Bushwick Hospital increased the size of its board of directors from nine to fifteen members in 1903; and by 1904 the board president, Charles Jewett, claimed that "the year has demonstrated the wisdom of enlarging the Board."[31] Added board members were far more lucrative than bake sales.

Older trustees selecting new members were faced with the problem of finding persons wealthy and notable enough to become trustees. Socially prominent families like the Schermerhorns, the Gerrys, the

Frothinghams, the Lows, the Roosevelts, and the Pierreponts were generally unwilling to extend their patronage beyond the institutions to which they were already committed. Furthermore, even the more established hospitals experienced a shortage of board members as older trustees died and others left for more central locations in the larger city.[32] This meant that the competition for the old family patronage that was available became intense.

Unable to draw new members from the older merchant families who traditionally served as stewards to charity facilities, hospital boards turned to the new group of businessmen, some of whom were at the head of the move toward industrialization. Because these men had few of the long-standing ties to New York and Brooklyn that characterized older trustees, they did not share in the tradition of paternalism toward the poor in their community. Their interest in hospitals was based more on their desire to exercise financial expertise and rescue the hospitals than on any interest in the moral and social reformation of patients. Though there were questions about the social position of some of these businessmen, it was at least hoped that they could help out in a difficult financial situation.

Small and struggling Brooklyn hospitals were quickly forced to turn to the local business community for board candidates. At Bushwick, for instance, the president announced that "several businessmen of East Brooklyn, well-known for their commercial eminence, accepted positions on the Board." Among these men were H. C. Bohack, owner of a number of produce stores in the Bushwick area, and N. H. Levi, a local businessman. This group, not having the social credentials of the older members of the board, were "chosen for their eminence in public affairs." As the older trustees saw it, "the business interests of the hospital could not more effectively be safeguarded, nor its prospects better assured," than by directly involving these businessmen.[33]

Older hospitals soon added prominent businessmen and industrialists to the socially important trustees who already appeared at the board meetings. Harold Pratt, an industrialist whose income was derived from Greenpoint oil refineries and from his father's close association with John D. Rockefeller, became president of Brooklyn Hospital in 1914. Abraham Abraham, the founder of Abraham and Straus, one of the city's largest department stores, became the first president of the Jewish Hospital of Brooklyn when it was organized in 1904.[34]

These new trustees brought with them innovative ideas about managing the hospitals' finances. As the larger society began to feel the influence of businessmen and efficiency-minded reformers, so too did hospital boards.[35] Believing in efficiency, bureaucracy, and cost accounting, these recently recruited businessmen sought to implement management and administrative procedures that, in fact, promised solvent and viable health institutions.

Nonetheless, the ability of these new trustees to manage finances was not sufficient to forestall conflict with the older trustees whose perspective was so different. Early in the Progressive period, most trustees saw their institutions as simply a charity for the poor. They perceived themselves as "the almoners of public and private charity" whose task was to reform the character of their patients as much as to manage finances.[36] Not until late in the Progressive era did they find it necessary to defend their position as guardians of the poor from attacks by the newer trustees who thought that board members should function as financial managers. In protest against the call of newer trustees for changes in accounting procedures, reforms in hospital organization, and closer inspection of the patients' ability to pay, the president of Lutheran Hospital exclaimed, "Our hospital work is a work of mercy. It is not a business."[37] The dialogue between trustees as reported in annual reports and trustees' minutes became increasingly tense and argumentative. The conflict between older members who advocated familiar laissez–faire methods of hospital financing and new trustees who advocated planned, long-term financial security and freedom from debt was particularly pronounced in the older facilities. Longtime board members found it difficult to view debt as a problem. For them a slight debt had always been a way to prove the neediness of the hospital and its patients.

In institutions first organized for new immigrants during the Progressive era, the conflict was less pronounced. New boards of trustees were actually created by businessmen, with only a rare member from an established merchant family. The Jewish Hospital of Brooklyn, for instance, was begun in 1903 ostensibly as a hospital run along business principles. "Even charitable institutions, however laudable and worthy, should be conducted on sound business principles," announced Abraham Abraham, president of the board. "The principal reason why so many charitable institutions are in financial difficulty," he observed, "is the fact that they permit their enthusiasm to sway their judgment and this condition, as a rule, can be charged to a wrong beginning." Abraham vowed to avoid the financial crises overtaking other hospitals. "The reports of our various charitable activities," he remarked, ". . . all ring . . . the one 'leit motif' and the one refrain: Appeal upon appeal to the public to help pay off large mortgages and other indebtedness." Abraham resolved that the Jewish Hospital would not repeat this pattern. "I commend the wisdom of your Board," he said as he spoke to

Brooklyn's Jewish community, "in their fixed determination not to run in debt."[38]

Abraham and other trustees of this newest hospital did not feel that careful business management needed to conflict with the hospital's caring function. From their perspective, care could be provided only if the hospital were financially stable. But for many trustees reared in the older ideals of stewardship for the poor, the idea of a hospital that was not as poor as its clients was incongruous; hospitals were, by definition, in debt and dependent on charitable contributions. When forced by circumstance to accept the guidance and reforms of a new class of businessmen and industrialists, some trustees were vehement in their objections. "Past generations of noble men who have built up the great fabric of American benevolence . . . lament such a radical change in American charitable methods," noted Frank Tucker, vice-president of a major New York insurance company, in his review of suggestions for changes in hospital financing. Some trustees even objected to calls for large, permanent endowments or community chests to provide stable income for all of New York City's hospitals. Essentially they feared any changes that might disrupt their traditional roles as financial guardians of their particular hospitals. W. Emlen Roosevelt of New York's Roosevelt Hospital summed up the views of many older trustees when he objected to the idea of a community chest on the grounds that hospitals should continue to "rely upon the charity of the wealthy men of New York for additional endowment."[39]

Though the desire and determination of many trustees was to remain the sole providers for their respective institutions, in reality they lacked the means to resist the financial pressures that lent credence to the position of the newer businessman-turned-trustee. As Tucker observed, these older trustees were "only men and not all [were] wizards of finance." He knew they were without solutions when he said, "They must have more [money]," and asked rhetorically, "but how can it be gotten?"[40] No longer could a few wealthy men defray mounting hospital deficits.[41] However the older trustees felt about the new businessmen on their boards, they had no choice but to consider the question posed by these newcomers: How will hospitals survive now that philanthropy is not enough?

The larger hospitals with substantial endowments and investments in bonds, stocks, and land had several options for solving their financial crises in the post-Depression years. At New York Hospital, for instance, the board of governors recognized that they were running up substantial deficits and, by 1900, had a total floating debt of over $650,000, which was growing "at the rate of from $75,000 to $100,000 per annum."[42] In response, the governors formed a committee to investigate the ways by which the solvency of their institution could be guaranteed. Whereas many of the smaller hospitals faced immediate bankruptcy, the growing deficits for this hospital posed a long-term problem calling for long-term solutions.

New York Hospital, by the early years of the twentieth century, had enormous financial resources at its disposal. It owned stocks and bonds on various railroads valued at over $700,000, it owned property valued at over $450,000, and it had savings accounts at three major banks of over $1 million.[43] This hospital hardly depended upon raffles, Christmas parties, cake sales, or receipts from occasional lectures as an important source of income. When its supporters donated, they donated substantial amounts. For instance, in addition to leaving the hospital land in the "Bathgate" section in the Bronx, Charles Bathgate Beck, also gave $359,000 to the hospital in the eight years between 1899 and 1907.[44]

When the hospital's crisis became obvious, the committee suggested a variety of remedies. The hospital could sell land, increase income from the paying patient building, or reform internal management practices. William Ryan, a prominent public accountant, was brought into the hospital by the trustees to analyze its accounting practices, management, and organization and to advise the trustees on the best methods for cutting costs. Ryan suggested a number of reforms, ranging from double-entry accounting for patient receipts in the outpatient and in-house departments to the formation of a central purchasing and supply department that would store and keep an inventory of all hospital supplies and the keeping of a record of costs by department. He also suggested the introduction of a receiving clerk and a storekeeper who would be in charge of a card-filing and inventory system.[45] By 1903 these basic management reforms were shown to pay valuable dividends to the institution. From January through March, the monthly expenditures for the hospital steadily decreased from $23,516 to $18,519 per month, a fact that did not go unnoticed by the trustees.[46]

The question of charging for services

Brooklyn's small hospitals had fewer alternatives for handling the financial crisis than did those institutions in Manhattan which had more access to wealthy benefactors. When the Memorial Hospital made the mistake of expanding its services in 1894 at the start of the Depression, "they had an uphill and hopeless struggle from the day [it] was opened . . . The efforts of the [hospital's] managers were futile. Disas-

August, 1917
Vol. IV, No. 1

HOSPITAL MANAGEMENT

608 S. Dearborn
Street,
Chicago

Published in the Interest of Executives in Every Department of Hospital Work
Entered as second class matter May 14, 1917, at the post office at Chicago, Ill., under the act of March 3, 1879.

It Takes a Pretty Good Bridge to Stand Up These Days

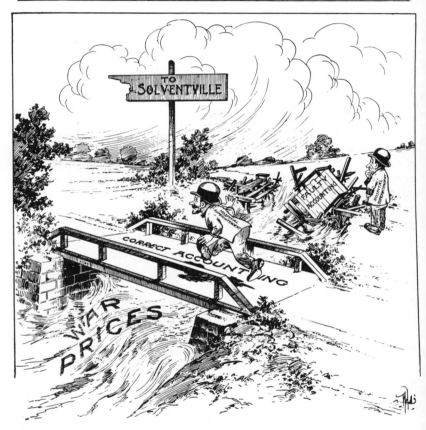

Some institutions developed new tools for financial management. In the face of growing costs, accentuated in this case by the inflation resulting from World War I, administrators were once again admonished to reform their accounting procedures if they wanted to get across the bridge to "Solventville."

ter after disaster overtook them until burdened with debt the Memorial Hospital Association had to succumb."[47] Until city government began to object, small hospitals could ask for stipends to support their
work. Under pressure from homeopathic physicians and lay persons,
the recently consolidated City of New York was called upon to take
over the Brooklyn Homeopathic Hospital in 1900. The *Brooklyn Daily
Eagle* recounted the unusual terms of the agreement: "When the details
came up, it was found that there were $70,000 debts on the hospital,
which the city was called upon to assume." After a period of renova-
tion, the city reopened the facility as the Cumberland Hospital. Several
institutions, such as the Memorial Hospital for Women and Children,
the Homeopathic Maternity Hospital, Eastern District Hospital, and
Williamsburg Hospital, were forced to close, consolidate, or join the
municipal hospital system during the Progressive era.[48]

Those institutions unable to reform their management practices, to
attract increased philanthropic support or donations, or to gain additional financial support from the city, were often forced to choose
between decreasing their services or passing costs on to their patients.
Generally the choice to decrease services was made before a move
toward charging patients. In 1894 the president of Brooklyn Nursery
and Infants' Hospital remarked: "Early last winter it became apparent
that something must be done to procure immediate pecuniary relief. A
cruel fact stared us in the face . . . We had been rolling up a debt which
there seemed no way of paying off." He noted that the hospital's
income had not kept pace with expenditures and that they "had come
to the cross-roads." After careful study, "our advisors decided that . . .
we should limit our inmates to a number which would keep our expenses down to a point commensurate with our resources." The Nursery and Infants' Hospital faced the same problem as did the other
institutions, and in the face of possible bankruptcy they cut down on
service to needy patients. "This was a hard lesson for us to learn – to
turn away so many needy, helpless ones," lamented the president.[49]

Some institutions felt that they had no choice but to begin charging
patients. Traditionally, charity institutions had refrained from charging any significant amount for the services patients received because it
was assumed that most were too poor to pay for their own care. Only
in rare circumstances, when travelers or others deemed capable of
payment were admitted, would substantial charges be made. Generally
a token payment was accepted from patients if their moral well-being
was judged to require it. Payment, like cleaning, aiding, or nursing
others in the hospital, was considered a way for the patient to meet his
obligation to a particular institution and was meant to develop the

patient's moral character as much as to support the hospital. For most hospitals, these payments were only a modest source of income.

The implementation of more rigorous payment schemes for patients was made somewhat easier by the fact that the Depression had already upset the internal workings of the hospital. Because the Depression left more people out of work, sick, and in need of the hospital's services, the administration had a tendency to move patients through the hospital more quickly than in the past: "The rapidity with which our work goes may be judged by the fact that the average stay of our patients was only about twenty-three days. This was three days less than during the preceding year," noted one hospital superintendent.[50] "Our wards and rooms are frequently crowded," complained the same superintendent. "Increasing service to the sick is made possible, under the limitation of stationary facilities, only by shortening their stay with us." This superintendent observed that "criticisms will be heard" because of such a policy, but added that "our justification is invariably in the fact that more needy persons are waiting to come."[51] At Methodist Hospital the average length of stay declined precipitously during the Depression years from 25.87 days per patient in 1893 to 18.08 days per patient in 1899. During these years, what had been a slow drop became a veritable plunge in average length of stay at Brooklyn Hospital – from 29.4 days in 1895 to 20.1 days in 1900 (see Table 3).[52]

This drastic drop in the length of patient stays eroded the personal and paternalistic relationship that had previously existed between trustees and patients. Hospitals no longer provided leisurely homelike care but hurried patients through in great numbers. Little time could be spent in establishing a relationship with patients – let alone reforming them morally. Because patients were not around long enough to do cleaning or nursing in exchange for their care, token payments took on a real significance. The short stays that deprived trustees of a personal relationship to patients also made it a bit easier to charge these patients when the hospital needed money.

Sometimes the number of paying patients was increased at the expense of those who had formerly been charity patients. "Notwithstanding [the] many and delightful entertainments which have earned for the Hospital a considerable sum, we still find our treasury more than empty," declared the secretary of the Memorial Hospital. "We, to lessen expense, are restricting our staff in the admission of *free patients*." According to the hospital's income, "we should be restricted to the care of *but ten* free patients"; instead, "we have had at times *about fifty*."[53] George Fisher, president of the Board of the Eastern District Dispensary and Hospital, had voiced a similar view years earlier when he said that it was "quite true that there is no limit to the amount of charitable work to be done, but there is a limit to our resources, and we should study these resources and conform our expenditures to them."[54]

The choice to restrict service for nonpaying patients and to seek patients who could pay often meant that the facilities formerly used for free patients were transformed into the kinds of rooms that would attract paying patients. "Further space in the wards must be prepared for the [paying] service if we wish to further increase our income from this source," declared John E. Leech and Edward Kidder, the vice-president and secretary of the Brooklyn Hospital in 1899.[55] By the spring of 1900, a "special committee of the Trustees" had made "a recommendation that the accommodations for pay patients be increased." With the death of the hospital's president, James H. Frothingham (whose father had also once been president), John Leech succeeded to the presidency. In his first annual statement he called "for some energetic action" to meet increased deficits.[56] By 1902 it was reported that the "trustees have decided to shut out part of the charity patients. It has been decided to keep expenditures down in this way, the hospital having, in the past, attempted to do more charity work than it could afford."[57] The fact that trustees began to see the patient as a source of income was reflected in the growing percentage of the hospital's budget derived from paying patients. In 1892, only 16 percent of the Brooklyn Hospital's budget came directly from paying patients. By 1900, the percentage had nearly doubled, and by the Banker's Panic of 1907, paying patients were contributing over 45 percent of the hospital's budget (see Figure 5).

Other hospitals also consciously turned to paying patients as an important source of income. As early as 1890, the Methodist Hospital had recognized the importance of the paying patient when its superintendent declared that the "completion of the Central Building would . . . furnish us with far more suitable apartments" for private patients. "It would also add some thousands of dollars to our income," he noted, "by rendering available a dozen or more private rooms for which invalids having means would gladly pay handsome prices."[58]

Hospital after hospital began to note increased dependence upon paying patients. As the hospitals' financial security was increasingly tied to the moneys derived from patients, charging fees became more and more of a necessity. Brooklyn's small Lutheran Hospital, for instance, noted that its financial stability was "brought about to a great extent by [its] many patients." It was true that the "congregation also sent gifts, but not as many as one could expect."[59] In 1894 the Methodist Hospital acknowledged that "the income from . . . private patients has aided very materially in maintaining the 'free work' of the institution."[60] Others flatly declared, "Additional income must be had, and that can come only from pay patients."[61] Abraham Abraham clearly stated that patient payments would maintain the Jewish Hospital's financial stability: "While our main purpose will be the operation of a charity hospital, we can devote one wing to pay patients. In this way, we can obtain sufficient revenue from the well-to-do to make up the deficiency for the running expenses and at the same time, not overlook the main purpose of the undertaking, the charity patient."[62]

This movement toward accepting the patient as a significant factor in hospital financing made it necessary for trustees and administrators to convince people that their institutions were still charities, because the fact became less obvious. When the president of Lutheran Hospital's board of trustees tried to maintain that his facility was "a work of mercy . . . not a business," he was forced to acknowledge that some "might be of a different opinion on account of our charges for care and room."[63] The president of the Bushwick Hospital declared in 1907, "We are not in hospital work to make money, but to help the sick and the suffering."[64]

The change from a predominantly "free" institution to a "pay" facility was not accomplished easily or without sacrifice. As will be discussed, there was *not* a ready, willing, and able cohort of new clients to whom the hospital could turn as a source of richer paying patients. Those who could pay did not see the hospital as an appropriate place for health care and chose to be treated at home. Not until later in the century would the hospital begin to shed the stigma attached to it by virtue of its status as a social service for needy people, and only then would wealthier patients come to the hospital. In the meantime, the patients being charged by the hospital were the poor and often struggling working-class people of the city who had formerly received care for a nominal charge.

The shift to a paying service also meant that these clients who were once considered worthy candidates for charity and moral reform came to be viewed as the perpetrators of the financial crisis afflicting institutions. A "fruitful cause for the annual deficiency in the hospitals," remarked Ogden Chisholm of New York's Babies' Hospital, "is the large number of free patients." Chisholm remarked that there were "thousands of people each year [some] of whom could pay something." He concluded that "if hospital patients had more honor and pride, I do not think there would be any large deficiency."[65] Administrators, angry perhaps that they could no longer afford to provide free services, began to resent the very people their hospitals had been organized to serve.

In the waning years of the Progressive era, prominent members of New York's Taylor Society and the Harvard Medical Club listened to a paper on the reorganization of Brooklyn's hospitals. This paper, delivered by Robert L. Dickinson, a prominent Brooklyn physician and leader in the birth control movement, stimulated serious discussion among persons in the hospital administration and larger scientific management movements. Dickinson captured the growing feeling that hospital work was no longer a charitable enterprise but was now a business whose work could be rationalized in the same way as that of other commercial enterprises.[66] Scientific management was to have only an indirect effect on the various phases of hospital work for many years, but Ernest Codman's comment at the conclusion of the paper reflected the fears and concerns of many involved in hospital work. "Our charitable hospitals have become businesses," this prominent surgeon noted, "and are . . . wolves in sheep's clothing."[67]

The idea of "hospital-as-business" was shocking and threatening to hospital trustees and charity workers who had organized, managed, and financed older charity facilities. They feared that the substantial changes in the hospital's role and function caused by the financial crisis during the previous decades had seriously undermined the integrity of the charity hospital. Though changes in financing helped hospitals to weather the Depression, those which survived were very different from what they had been. The difference is clearly reflected in the position of the trustees. In the past a small number of trustees had run the hospital largely out of their feeling of personal responsibility to the institution and its patients. With the financial crisis of the Depression, boards expanded and were forced to focus more on financial management than on caring. These larger boards were often composed of people from a wider range of social classes, and the goals of businessmen on the board tended to conflict with those of the older trustees. Paternalist notions of caring often were challenged by the principles of sound business.

The dependence of the hospital on direct patient payment also changed the basic relationship between trustees and their patients. Because some patients were now buying services, they could make demands as they never had before. The hospital, on the other hand, had to focus on reforming its internal organization and catering to those doctors who might bring in paying patients.

3   Social class and hospital care

Because hospital trustees could no longer depend primarily on private benefactors to support their institutions and were instead forced to begin charging patients significant sums, it became necessary to organize and present the hospital to the public in a new way. If patients were to be encouraged to pay for services, the hospitals would have to offer them something different from the services provided at minimal or no charge to the indigent. Some trustees and hospital spokesmen began to organize distinct services for different classes of the population – sometimes separate services within a single institution, and sometimes entirely separate institutions for those who could pay and those in need of charity care.

Once separate private services were introduced, it became necessary to convince the merchants, white-collar workers, and skilled craftsmen who might be expected to use them that hospital care was superior to the treatment they had traditionally received at home, sometimes with the aid of private physicians and private-duty nurses. Accordingly, hospitals began to offer amenities like private and semiprivate rooms, private nurses, better food, and pleasant accommodations for those patients willing to pay the price. But more was necessary to attract to the hospital people who had long received private medical care in their homes. Hospital representatives began to advertise their improved services and also to encourage public newspaper reports from patients convinced of the superiority of hospital care. Often these reports portrayed the hospital as nothing more than a "hotel for rich invalids."

Although initially these efforts seemed to promise the presence of a wealthier clientele who would use the private services, in the end only a small number of upper- or middle-class patients actually came to the hospital as a result of these efforts. Ultimately, trustees would see that only by forging an alliance with private practitioners who would bring their patients to the hospital would the long-standing prejudices against the charity hospital be dispelled. Only then would the hospital administration be able to count on full use of the private services and a substantial increase in income received directly from patients.

The internal restructuring of the facility would ultimately result in the kind of institution we have with us today, one in which services

HOSPITAL MANAGEMENT

Vol. VII, No. 3.
October, 1919

417 S. Dearborn
Street,
Chicago

Published in the Interest of Executives in Every Department of Hospital Work

The Class in Hospital Designing

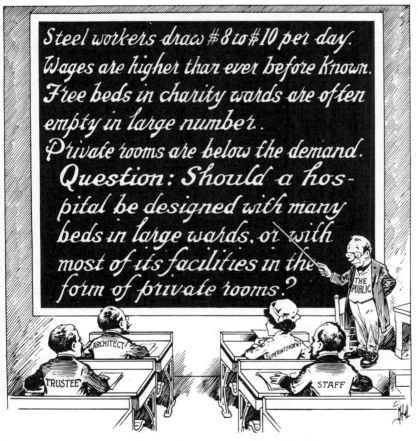

As late as 1919 the journal *Hospital Management* still sought to convince trustees, architects, superintendents, and the hospital staff that there was a demand for a greater number of private rooms. This was still not obvious to many across the country.

are bought and care is often seen as a commodity. As administrators began to inspect them and investigate their financial capabilities, patients were gradually made to feel that they should pay for their care. But a more important method of guaranteeing payment was to improve the quality of the paid services. Grades of service and different kinds of amenities were introduced into a previously one-class facility as a means of inducing patients to pay for care. Soon charity services were seen as degrading in comparison to the paid services, and those who used them as immoral or lazy. Although it was largely the working class who used the hospital throughout the Progressive era, the changing financial base and the changing goals of the institution profoundly altered the hospital's previous charitable intent. As one contemporary observer remarked, it was "obvious that there can be no very great increase in income from [paying patients] unless the accommodations for the rich are increased at the expense of space allotted now to those who can pay a small amount and those who cannot pay at all."[1] The development of the new noncharity hospital demanded the internal reorganization and rebuilding of the older charity hospital and the abandonment of its commitment to the poor.

The differentiation of hospital services

There was much question about the necessity, and even the morality, of the move away from charity services. Nonetheless, some public officials and administrators pressed for the widespread introduction of patient payments as the salve that would soothe the wound of growing deficits. As Homer Folks, the commissioner of public charities, argued during the 1904 conference on the financial crisis of the city's hospitals: "A diligent effort to collect from all [independent hospital] patients not wholly destitute some part of the cost of their care, might result in considerable diminution of the deficits."[2] Because the city was expanding its public hospital system and its per capita, per diem hospital reimbursement scheme, public officials felt that the needs of the poor were being met. In fact, the city felt far less dependent on charity hospitals to care for the poor than they had in the past. They consequently felt free to try to convince administrators in independent charity hospitals that their patients were nonindigent and able to pay for at least part of their hospital care.[3]

Although some trustees and administrators of the city charity hospitals objected to the suggestion that hospitals should make a habit of charging patients for services that had always been considered charitable, others quickly embraced this suggestion and sought reform of what were considered sloppy inspection procedures. Sidney Goldstein, an administrator at Mount Sinai Hospital in Manhattan, lamented the inadequacy of the prevailing system of hospital admission procedures, and noted that there was "absent almost completely any endeavor to discover the patient's ability to contribute toward his maintenance or treatment."[4] He and other administrators thought that they could locate patients capable of paying by merely tightening the procedures used to determine ability to pay. But others thought that more was needed. So long as free services were the same as services for which people paid, and so long as no stigma was attached to the use of these services, people would not be motivated to pay and might very well lie in order to continue using free wards. Several observers recommended that the pay and charity services of hospitals be differentiated according to *types* and *quality* of services. In general, it was suggested that the paying services should consist of private rooms, smaller wards, and better-quality food. Paying patients would be treated by their private physicians, and those using the charity services by the younger house staff.

In a paper read before the New York Medical Society in 1901, one hospital-based physician proposed a strict separation of the indigent and the paying patient. He argued "that people who have money and are willing to pay for a bed in a public hospital should not be thrust into a ward in companionship with a pauper; that the pauper had no right to share in their treatment and, further, that the criminal pauper [had] sacrificed all rights other than what justice and humanity deemed should be his."[5] To this observer, as long as the services provided in the hospital were undifferentiated, there would be little incentive for those who could pay for their care to do so. Administrative determinants were inadequate for clearly differentiating patients able to pay from the truly indigent. With the institution of separate services, patients would be forced to differentiate services by choosing that level of care they could best afford.

The most concrete implication of this desire to separate patients according to economic class and ability to pay for services was the widespread agreement that new kinds of facilities had to be built for different classes of the population. During the early twentieth century, what had been a relatively small contingent of private services was rapidly expanded. In larger hospitals such as New York, Roosevelt, and St. Luke's, private pavilions were constructed to house paying patients. In smaller facilities that lacked the funds to build new additions, some wards were converted from large open spaces into private and semi-private rooms. Floors and even wards were divided into separate areas for "free" and "pay" patients.

The growing interest of hospital administrators and physicians in private room and ward patients clearly threatened the charity functions of the hospital. Some directly involved in providing services in the older charity facilities thought that this segregation of patients according to class constituted a crude and immoral introduction of business principles into the charity facility. When New York's Roosevelt Hospital distributed a circular calling attention to its newly opened private rooms and private pavilion, editorial response was negative. The *Trained Nurse and Hospital Review*, the most important nursing journal of the day, noted that the "circular all through savors of the modern business advertising proclamation . . . just as Wanamaker advertises a store opening and a new stock of goods." The editorial objected even more strenuously to the new direction the hospital was taking as it switched from a charity facility to a voluntary institution dependent on paying patients. "Here is a great public hospital, endowed richly, consecrated to philanthropy and benevolence, using the funds left in charity's name to equip private rooms . . . for those able to pay the price," commented the editor. "In the spirit of fairness, and in the name of charity . . . we ask, 'Is it right?' " The editors clearly objected to the apparent take-over of sections of this hospital by those able to "pay the price."[6]

Others directly and indirectly involved in medical care sought an even more drastic reorganization of services. Some called for the strict separation of paying and free patients in entirely different institutions. In a 1905 editorial called "Abolish the Hospital Grafter," the *Journal of the American Medical Association* suggested that the "abuse" of hospital facilities by those able to pay for their care could be stopped only by the differentiation of facilities according to social class. The "absolute segregation of charity patients from pay patients" was necessary to stop misuse of services, the editorial declared. "Those who really have no means will perforce go to the genuine charity hospitals, while few of those who have any income will sink their pride so far as to enter an institution patronized by none but the destitute." The editorial remarked that when "the only alternative is a pay hospital where none are treated free, the deed is done. So long as rich and poor are treated under one roof, the well-to-do will not scruple at getting free treatment if they can as no stigma attaches to residence in an institution where many pay their way."[7]

The *New York Times* echoed this opinion, but did so from a distinctly different perspective. In a stinging editorial in 1904 entitled "The Problems of the Hospitals," the *Times* called for a total reorganization of the municipal and private hospital system. The *Times* distinguished two groups then demanding hospital care: the traditional poor and indigent recipients of hospital treatment, and a new class of wealthier patients who had begun to use the hospital much as they might use a hotel.[8]

The editorial identified a number of causal factors in this shift to the hospital as the focus of much health care. First, it noted that former prejudices concerning the hospital were waning; second, it observed that new standards of medicine demanded centralized sanitary institutions. But most important, the *Times* saw that housing conditions in the rapidly expanding city had created a need for a new institution for wealthy clients. As large numbers of the city's population moved into apartments, tenements, and hotels, the paper remarked, the cramped conditions of such facilities mitigated against care for the ill, and removal from the home setting became necessary. The *Times* hypothesized that the hospital was becoming a convenience for white-collar and middle-class groups, an "invalid's hotel," and not a necessity for the poor alone. "Hotels and apartments answer very well for all the purposes of comfortable living under the conditions of normal health," the *Times* commented, "but they are inconvenient places in which to be sick, offering very little opportunity for quiet or privacy."[9] Wealthier clients began to usurp hospital beds in independent facilities, thereby limiting the poor's access to those beds.

The hospital's changing function, the *Times* felt, increased the need for stricter separation of the wealthy and poor patients. One institution, it was maintained, could not serve both groups adequately. What was needed was a "general reorganization of our hospital system . . . The present tendency is to make it increasingly difficult for all who need hospital accommodations as charity patients to secure admissions to the wards. The beds are filled and the facilities . . . taxed by those who use the hospitals merely as conveniences."[10] The editorial called for the strict separation of the social classes into distinct institutions, in order to guarantee that service for the indigent would not be neglected in attempts to please the wealthy.

The *Times* also argued that a number of organizational and financial imperatives demanded a strict separation of the wealthy and the poor. As long as the paying and free patient were serviced in the same facility, the business interests of the hospital would conflict with its charitable goals. Furthermore, the presence of wealthy patients raised the administrative costs of the hospital. The "scale of administrative expenses demanded in the case of what is in fact a hotel for rich invalids or those in comfortable circumstances is perhaps out of proportion to the requirements of a charity hospital." The *Times* observed that the integration of patient classes undermined the image of the hospital as a charity. Philanthropists, observing that there were wealthy and poor in the same institution, might mistakenly assume that the institution was no longer in need of donations. At a time of severe financial strain, such a critique appeared justified and threatening. Because "invalid hotels" should be self-sustaining and run on "sound business principles," the *Times* editorial noted, an "endeavor to maintain a dual character [does] not appeal to philanthropists as inviting objects of bequests and benefaction."[11]

Whereas the *Times* and the *Journal of the American Medical Association* argued for a separation of services, others went a step further and argued for "two classes of hospitals." F. R. Sturgis proposed that there should be public institutions managed by the city for the care of the sick poor and a set of private institutions "distributed in various parts of the city, for the reception of persons of means, strangers resident in New York City, and others who require hospital attendance." The key distinctions between the patients in the public and the private systems would be their ability to pay for room and board. The "private hospitals," Sturgis declared, "shall decline to take any patients who are unable to at least pay board," whereas the indigent "shall be looked after by the city." Sturgis explained "in plain English" that "the [private] hospital would be a medical hotel"; the municipal hospitals "would be reserved for the poor alone."[12]

The advantages of this plan were obvious to Sturgis. First, a neat division of labor between the municipal and private hospitals guaranteed hospital services to the poor as well as the wealthy. The city would take over care for the indigent, and the private facilities would provide services to the white-collar worker and others able to pay. Second, this system would integrate the "hotel hospitals" into the larger economic system by forcing them to respond to more general laws of supply and demand. The weak institutions would no longer be able to survive because of philanthropic donations, but would sink or float according to their appeal to wealthier clients. This, in turn, would serve to centralize and consolidate an otherwise disorganized and diffuse hospital system. Sturgis declared "that there are more hospitals than are necessary," and too many hospitals "duplicate their work . . . and so intensify the evil which must result from an improper division of labor." His plan was a version of the Darwinian notion of "survival of the fittest" to hospital organization: "If there are too many which cannot be supported, . . . it is evident that [some] must go out of business." In his more benign moments, Sturgis suggested that the "hospitals get together, and decide which ones shall continue in business, and which shall not."[13]

Many administrators, officials, and doctors in New York agreed that there were too many hospitals – at least, too many small financially unstable and nonprestigious institutions whose presence tarnished the overall image of hospital work. What was needed, according to the most powerful and important spokesmen in the health system, was a centralized and bureaucratized hospital system that would efficiently service all classes of the city's population in socially distinct facilities. The *Times* and Sturgis advocated such a system, one that would concentrate power in the hands of the largest, best-equipped, and most powerful institutions in the city. The public hospital system would be primarily responsible for providing charity services to indigent and dependent hospital patients, whereas the private and independent hospitals would be increasingly tied to the business of attracting and servicing the paying patient. The creation of this system of separate, but not necessarily equal, facilities would require massive intervention and manipulation: Only a reversal in policy would get the independent facilities to revert to caring only for charity clients; and the construction of new facilities for the "wealthier invalid" would require a massive outlay of funds.

The *Times* and Sturgis were both recommending that the hospital for the nonpaying laborer be separate from the facility for the white-collar worker. That "the same central idea" came "from two such distinguished and diverse sources" led *Charities*, the Charity Organization Society's journal, to survey the opinions of superintendents in Manhattan's largest hospitals. First, superintendents were asked to classify their patients as charity patients, patients of moderate means, or well-to-do patients. Second, they were asked to identify the class they considered in greatest need of hospital services. Third, they were asked whether they favored strict segregation of paying and charity patients in separate "buildings or institutions, or . . . the present plan of caring for all classes in the same institution." The final task for the superintendents was to surmise the possible effect on donations and legacies of a plan to separate patients and to judge whether any "hospital [could be] self-supporting without donations and legacies."[14]

The results of this survey were surprising. First, nearly all of the superintendents agreed with George P. Ludlam of the prestigious New York Hospital that "the greatest need . . . is for the non-paying patients." James Lathrop, at Roosevelt, echoed this opinion, noting that "there is no doubt in my own mind that the 'greatest need for increased provision in New York' is for that class of patients who are unable to pay anything, or the nominal sum of $1 or $1.50 per day." C. Irving Fisher of Presbyterian and George C. Glover at St. Luke's concurred.[15]

Second, none of the five hospital superintendents interviewed agreed with the *Times* and Sturgis that there should be separate hospitals for the poor and the nonindigent. "The division of hospitals into the two classes proposed and their distinct separation seems impracticable," noted Ludlam. This plan, he argued, "would pre-suppose that the pay hospitals would be self-supporting . . . dependent upon the income from patients," an assumption that he found untenable. Rather, the "separation [within the hospital] of patients able to pay liberally for their accommodation and treatment from those able to pay only a nominal rate, or not at all, is quite proper." Separation according to social class, Ludlam pointed out, was an accepted tenet in many areas of American life. Such separation might be accomplished by placing one group of patients "in a separate building in the same plant, or in a part of the building thoroughly shut off by itself, or in a separate hospital maintained exclusively for that class of patients."[16]

The superintendents not only disagreed that separate institutions were necessary to distinguish between services, but also regarded strict separation of patients *within* the same institution as a way to maintain the older paternalistic relationship between the hospital's benefactors and those on the charity wards. Those who received free care or who paid only part of their hospital bills could still be seen as receiving some sort of charity. Those patients who paid for all of their hospital care could be viewed as benefactors of the institution's charity service, much as if they had made a donation. "Only those are classed as 'private patients' who pay for separate rooms and for 'luxuries,' " Lathrop remarked. "For such there exists here a separate pavilion quite apart from the ward service." The "charitable work of the hospital," Lathrop maintained, was "in no sense interfered with nor diminished" by such a setup, for patrons were now patients within the same institution.[17]

Others also maintained that private patients were continuing the tradition of benevolent giving within the institution's walls. Glover of St. Luke's said that the "only patients who do not receive charity to some degree are those who occupy private rooms . . . and who pay the attending physician or surgeon a proper fee."[18] After all, as Lathrop remarked, "the existence of facilities for the care of 'private patients' makes it possible for the hospital to perform a greater charitable work than it could otherwise."[19] It became "the practice . . . in non-municipal hospitals [to devote] the profits that are realized from the care of full-pay or private room patients to the purpose of helping to defray the expense incurred in the care of non-paying patients, or patients for whom only partial payment is provided."[20] In effect, private patients came to be seen as the benefactors of ward patients, according to the theory "that private patients should be taken only at a profit, as a means of assisting in the maintenance of an institution primarily intended for the sick poor."[21]

Advertising the new hospital

For many hospitals there remained the problem of attracting patients who paid the full rate. Private patients, after all, were reluctant to come to institutions long associated with charity and working-class patients. The "private patient . . . comes to these institutions by election," pointed out a popular administrative text, "and therefore, the service received must be of a sufficiently high order to attract them."[22] Others noted that private patients were attracted only to certain rooms, "showing that the attractiveness of quiet, well-located and furnished rooms, with skillful physicians, surgeons, and nurses always in attendance, is rapidly removing the old-time prejudice against hospital treatment."[23] Though many thought there was a potential market for hospital-related services among wealthy apartment-dwelling clients, most recognized that these patients would be attracted only to institutions that catered to their special needs and interests: Appropriate services, reasonable costs and improved medical care were essential.

Inadequate service, high costs, and poor medical treatment in fact appeared responsible for the low occupancy of the new private patient pavilion opened in 1900 at New York Hospital. In September of 1901, George Ludlam, the hospital's superintendent, reported on this pavilion's first nine months of operation. He noted that the private rooms and paying wards of the Private Patient Building were grossly under-occupied during the year. Only 90 patients used the private rooms and 125 used the "intermediate wards," he reported. The "total number of [hospital] days [used] in the private rooms was 1879 – about 39 percent of the possible number, 4770," and "the total days in the intermediate wards was 3070 – about 32 percent of the possible number, 9540." This low occupancy rate translated into a poor financial return on investment, and Ludlam felt it wise to consider "whether any change in method would lead to a more satisfactory result."[24]

Ludlam's analysis of the reasons for the failure of the private service centered on a number of factors that limited the institution's appeal to wealthy patients. First, there was the cost of care in the institution. Like any other "hotel for rich invalids," the private service was in competition with other hospitals in the city for a relatively small number of patrons. Unfortunately for New York Hospital, "the present charges . . . are considerably higher than those made by other hospitals of similar standing. For instance, the prices at Roosevelt Hospital range from $25 to $75 per week; at the Presbyterian Hospital, from $25 to $40, and at the private hospital popularly called Dr. Bull's, from $25 to $75. Ours," Ludlam noted, "range from $25 to $100." He reported to the board of governors that "considerable comment has been made on the high rates charged by us. And the statement that patients have thus been deterred from coming, has been made by those whose opinions we value, with sufficient frequency to warrant the serious consideration of the subject." As might be done in any competitive industry, Ludlam recommended a series of pricing changes that would make his hospital marketable in the highly competitive hospital industry: "It would seem desirable to place more rooms at $25 per week, to increase the number of those ranging from $25 to $40, and to fix the highest price at $65." A corner room with a bath might be rented at $10 more per week. Although Ludlam and others still saw the private service as a profit-producing area of hospital work, they were forced to admit that their attempt to maximize profits by charging high room rates had backfired. Faced with resistance from consumers – in this case, wealthy patients – the hospital reduced its prices to competitive levels.[25]

Some trustees argued that more than haphazard reports and word of mouth was needed to convince middle-class people to come to the hospital. They declared that the absence of paying patients could be attributed "to the fact that the advantages offered by the pay service were not generally known," and recommended that "energetic efforts be made by advertising . . . the facilities."[26] By "inserting in the *Brooklyn Eagle* an advertisement calling the attention of the public to the advantages of the Hospital," they could perhaps persuade paying patients to throw off their long-standing prejudices against charity hospitals and see the advantages of the hospital ward in times of illness.[27]

Other trustees recognized that public prejudices against the hospital ran much deeper than many assumed. The public, or at least that portion of the public which could pay for hospital care, had a deep antipathy toward institutions traditionally associated with charity and pauperism. A committee of trustees at Brooklyn Hospital decided that

Vol. IX, No. 2
February, 1920

HOSPITAL MANAGEMENT

417 S. Dearborn
Street,
Chicago

Published in the Interest of Executives in Every Department of Hospital Work

Advertise to Them All

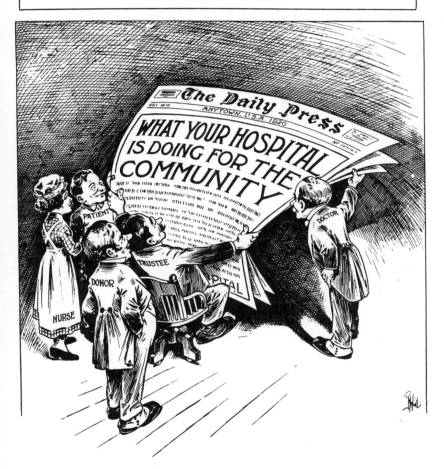

Public relations was increasingly important in changing the image of the hospital. Here *Hospital Management* suggests that the hospital should advertise its usefulness to the entire community.

what was really needed was a change in the image of the institution. By December 1894 George C. White and fellow trustees were pushing for a reeducation campaign "for the purpose of making the Hospital more widely known as a philanthropic and not a municipal Institution, and of educating the public in the advantages offered by the pay wards and private rooms."[28]

Brooklyn Hospital, originally named the Brooklyn City Hospital, had struggled for years with its identity as a charity institution whose name conveyed municipal sponsorship. In March 1883 the trustees chose to drop the word "City" from the corporation title. This was "deemed advisable because . . . the name conveyed the erroneous idea that it was a municipal corporation and supported by the city proper."[29] But in articles, on maps, and in common parlance, well into the 1890s, the Brooklyn Hospital was spoken of simply as "City Hospital."[30]

In the 1880s and early 1890s, the ramifications of being known as the "City Hospital" primarily affected philanthropic donation. Those who made small donations at Christmas or on other specific occasions might very well bypass an institution assumed to be publicly funded. "An impression has prevailed that this institution is a *public* charity, as distinguished from an *individual* undertaking, and that its support is derived from public funds," noted William Low, a member of one of Brooklyn's most prominent families and the president of this hospital. Low sought to correct this public perception by declaring that, contrary to popular belief, the hospital "depended from its beginning mainly upon private liberality for its continuance and support."[31]

The hospital's public image as a municipal facility had a wider and more troubling effect when trustees wished to attract paying patients. Patients were careful to avoid treatment in one of the city's almshouse hospitals. Brooklyn's Kings County Hospital and Manhattan's Bellevue Hospital had both developed in conjunction with the city's almshouses and prisons, so that the association of the prison, almshouse, and city hospital in the public mind tended to be strong enough to cause patients to seek other places for care. Trustees and administrators at Brooklyn Hospital found it imperative to convince the public that their institution was neither publicly sponsored nor a "City Hospital."

By December 3, 1894, White had convinced the committee and board to engage in an advertising campaign to inform the public of the hospital's nonmunicipal status and of "the advantages offered by the [hospital's] pay wards and private rooms."[32] A number of actions of varying importance were taken to advertise this information. A "handsome sign" was placed on the hospital's front lawn, and detailed "information about the hospital" was posted near the front gate. Large cards were printed and hung "in the larger stores, Lodge Rooms, factories, etc. to be accompanied by letters calling attention to the facilities offered in case of sickness or accidents." Such advertisements illustrated the fact that the trustees sought to attract factory workers, single clerks, and other workers who roomed in lodging houses.[33]

Though trustees were convinced that there was a ready market of clients who could afford to use paying services, they were vague in identifying this client population. In the eyes of the trustees, those "wealthy" enough to use the pay services ranged from independent merchants who could afford the expensive private rooms and suites to the clerk, the industrial worker, and the young, single seamstress who might pay for care in a private room or "paying ward." In addition to putting notices in lodging houses and factories, trustees advertised their services in the *Brooklyn Daily Eagle*, a newspaper that served an elite Protestant readership residing in the wealthy Brooklyn Heights area and in Park Slope. Throughout 1895, the trustees placed in the *Daily Eagle* "a carefully worded advertisement . . . once or twice a week" as a means of informing the community of the hospital's service.[34]

A change in the emphasis of the ads over time indicates the hospital's increasing interest in paying patients. The early ads, placed on the editorial page of the *Daily Eagle* (near advertisements for Scott's Emulsion for growing babies or Hood's Sarsparilla tonic), depicted the hospital as "Mainly supported by Voluntary Contributions" and noted that donations could be sent to the treasurer at Long Island Trust Company. But because the ads also listed the prices of rooms, including board, nursing, and medicines,[35] it was not always clear whether they were an appeal for philanthropic donations or for paying patients.

By the middle of the year, however, the ambiguity of the first advertisement was cleared up. The ads dropped the direct appeal for donations and emphasized the paying and private nature of available services. The words "free wards," and "children's wards" remained in lowercase letters in the ad, whereas the lines in capital letters read: "BEDS IN PAY WARDS, $7 PER WEEK. PRIVATE ROOMS FROM $12 to $25 PER WEEK." In addition, the public was informed that "trained nurses [were] furnished for private families." As this later advertisement indicates, the trustees clearly saw the salvation of the hospital in fees collected for services, rather than in philanthropic contributions.[36]

Somewhat different approaches were taken by New York's larger hospitals. Roosevelt Hospital circulated an advertisement describing the advantages of hospital care; Presbyterian Hospital printed a pamphlet with rates and descriptions of the private services; New York

Hospital printed a card giving room rates and rules regarding the new private patient pavilion. But New York Hospital's superintendent felt that more publicity might be necessary. "One other point may be deemed worthy of consideration," he told his board of governors: "Extensive, but judicious advertising" might solve the problem of low occupancy in the private service.[37]

It is not surprising, however, that there was a strong resistance to hospital care among many potential private patients. This resistance, based on popular conceptions of hospital care, was often starkly reported in the popular press and served as a strong reinforcement for existing prejudices. In 1900, for instance, two nurses at Bellevue Hospital were accused of poisoning a patient, and a newspaper editorial in the *Times* noted the broad consequences of the event. One was "the tendency which the revelation . . . will certainly have to revive the old horror of hospitals in general," the *Times* editor remarked. In recent years, this editorial stated, the "horror [of hospital care] had been fast diminishing" among all social classes.[38] But this scandal would "serve as an excuse for following the acknowledged, but not yet fully realized, delusion that love for the patient is the best equipment a nurse can possibly have," and would therefore prompt the ill to stay in their homes.[39]

Some of the stories of horrors in municipal and independent hospitals had a basis in truth. After all, it was only on August 27, 1887, that an order was issued prohibiting the use of one bed for two patients or two beds for every three patients when free beds were available. "I transmit the following," read a memo from Arthur Phillips, assistant secretary at the Department of Public Charities: "The Wardens of Bellevue and Charity Hospital [are to] see to it that in no case where there are empty beds in any ward of their institutions, shall they allow three patients to be placed in two beds, or two patients in any one bed, in any particular ward."[40]

At the Kings County Hospital, patients complained that the food "was not eatable and insufficient as well as badly prepared."[41] One patient who claimed that the food was "adequate" described the diet as consisting of coffee, bread, and butter at six o'clock in the morning; rice and milk at 9:30; a quart of soup made from meat and vegetables at noon; and gruel and milk at 4:30 in the afternoon. This patient stated that he was given "three heavy woolen blankets," though another correspondent complained that "he was only allowed one fourth of a blanket."[42]

Brooklyn's Methodist Episcopal Hospital, an independent charity facility, had its scandal as well. Maximino Casanova, a Cuban cigar dealer, reported that during his stay as a patient for seven weeks during the spring and summer of 1897, "the cruelty practiced by at least one of the nurses upon patients unnerved [him] to such an extent that when [he] finally left the hospital [his] health was poorer than it was when [he] entered." Declared Casanova, "I was a pay patient, . . . and was therefore given better treatment than those brought there on charity, but I could stand no longer the unpleasant sights and scenes in the hospital." He reported that he "saw an attendant hold a sick Pole down and poke his fingers in the man's eyes, simply because he could not understand English," and that "on another occasion this same attendant . . . grabbed an Italian patient and punched him in the ribs." Casanova also reported that an attendant "poured carbolic acid over a patient on the pretext that he wanted to kill vermin." On a further occasion, "another attendant slapped a paralyzed patient, and this so enraged two other patients in the ward that they got out of bed and chased the attendant." Hospital attendants, often drawn from the most alienated social groups, were noted for such mistreatment. Casanova's report went on to say that "it was impossible almost to get any attention in his ward. The attendants. . . played cards and other games, and when [he] would ask for some little attention [he] was frequently told that the nurse had no time to attend to [him]." Although the hospital's superintendent denied the claims, this report received attention in both the *Brooklyn Daily Eagle* and the *Times*.[43]

Although such complaints and editorials reinforced many people's distrust of the hospital, other articles began to appear offering glowing reports of service in the private wing. "I can go to St. Luke's and for $21 a week . . . I can have a private room, with board, medicines, medical and surgical attendance and a trained nurse constantly with me," declared one happy hospital patient in 1896. "There I am in a hotel, and I can have anything I want. Not only can my friends visit at any hour of the day or night, but they can be constantly with me. Indeed, they can rent the next room and live with me, as they could in any other hotel." This patient also recognized the economic advantage of residing in a hospital while receiving medical care. "Outside the hospital the nurse alone would cost me $25 a week . . . Inside I can pay more, if I desire a better room."[44] Another article, relating a "Girl's Hospital Experience," declared: "One is not quite in the swim nowadays if one has not had an operation performed . . . A hospital has nothing but pleasant associations for me, and you will never find me out of one again when I am ill."[45]

To attract the middle class, hospitals were increasingly portrayed as pleasant hotel-like places where people had freedom of movement and control over the activities of their day. "I reached the hospital, announced myself, and was shown upstairs to my room," a young lady recalled. "Then I began to have callers." The callers kept coming throughout the afternoon: First came the intern who took her family medical history. The superintendent followed, and then the doctor, who asked about her personal health. After this came the nurse. In the evening she read a good book and was "at liberty to enjoy myself as I pleased," reading until she was very sleepy. Even the food was delicious, for "they had a good chef"; she took delight in all the "delicacies of the season" served "in the daintiest way . . . in individual pots," and the china was "all most attractive."[46] The operation was painless and she immediately felt better and began to receive visitors.

Some hospitals were clearly intended to replicate the fanciest aspects of a good hotel. "In the New York Hospital," declared George Ludlam, its superintendent, "the new private patient pavilion . . . speaks for itself." Ludlam noted that the "new building has everything that modern sanitary knowledge can suggest and is like a great hotel, with its rooms prettily furnished with brass bedsteads, couches, Morris chairs, visiting desks, open fireplaces, double doors to each room, diet kitchens, and serving rooms." Furthermore, "there is pretty china for the service of meals, with every convenience."[47]

Some of the publicity for the hospital focused on the fact that the hospital relieved the family of a difficult emotional and financial burden and thereby eased the suffering of patient and family alike. "I don't believe there is any treatment more satisfactory in any kind of illness for one's own good or for that of the family," one hospital heroine remarked.[48] Not only was the hospital homelike, but it was better than home as far as family interference was concerned. "It can be put down as one of the advantages of a hospital that the relatives and friends do not take care of the patient," declared one hospital superintendent interviewed by the *Times*. "It is much better for them [patients] not to be under the care of any one who is over-concerned for them," he concluded.[49] As scientific medicine advanced, the expertise and professional distance of the doctor, not the love of relatives, came to characterize good care.

It was also pointed out that the cost of hospital care was low in comparison to similar services provided in the home. One young woman stated: "When one has had illness in the family, and knows how many towels and how many pieces of bed linen a good nurse feels are necessary for the welfare of her patient, and what trouble and expense it is to get it laundered, to say nothing of the other expenses – the cost of hospital treatment seems small."[50] Private-duty nursing, long the prerogative of wealthy patients who were treated in their home, was also shown to be very expensive. In the private rooms of the hospital, well-trained and supervised private nurses were available to patients at a lower cost than in private homes.[51] Because the hospitals provided both trained and student nurses, they could employ private nurses for shorter periods of time and for more defined tasks than could private citizens. Whereas many observers feel today that home care could reduce the costs of health care for patients who are now hospitalized, administrators in the early 1900s assumed the opposite: Hospitals were portrayed as a cost-saving device.

Changing notions of the nature of disease and of the means for controlling it also made the hospital seem superior to the home for care. First of all, protection from the common forms of infection that plagued surgical and medical patients demanded levels of cleanliness higher than were possible in many turn-of-the-century houses. Because Victorian tastes often tended toward clutter, it was difficult to maintain even a relatively germ-free environment. Hence the hospital, with its standing staff of nurses, cleaners, and launderers, was more efficient and less expensive than private care in the Victorian home.

The portrayal in the press of the hospital as hotel eventually succeeded in attracting some people to paying services. Once the public accepted the image of the private service as superior, few would choose to receive ward-based charity care if they could afford to pay. Rather than objecting to the image of ward services as inferior and sometimes dangerous, many hospital administrators saw that it could help to encourage patients to pay for private service.

The hospital-as-hotel image was, however, fraught with problems that were potentially destructive to the long-term acceptance of the hospital as a substitute for home as a place for care. The depiction of the hospital as loosely structured and even fun to be in contradicted the reality. Hospitals were tightly controlled institutions with a long history as agents of social rehabilitation. Administrators assumed that patients were to be isolated from the disease-producing and psychically debilitating environment outside the institution, and did not, in fact, allow them to have unlimited visitors, as the *Times* publicized. Most hospital administrators accepted that a greater degree of freedom was appropriate for the better-educated and wealthier clients, who were less in need of "social information," but too much latitude in the actions of any patient was considered detrimental, if only from the point of view of hospital routine. One hospital superintendent stated that if a patient "is richer . . . there are certain afternoons when his friends can visit," but that even private patients had to have limits: "We cannot

HOSPITAL MANAGEMENT

August, 1918
Vol. VI, No. 1

417 S. Dearborn Street, Chicago

Published in the Interest of Executives in Every Department of Hospital Work

"Signs of the Times" Point to the Hospital

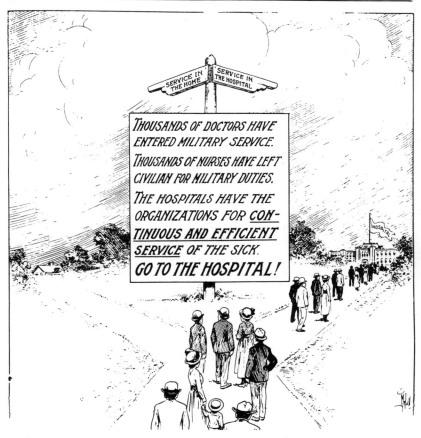

As late as 1918 most people still chose to stay at home for their medical care. The involvement of the United States in World War I, however, gave advocates of hospital services a new patriotic theme in their attempts to convince the middle class to use the hospital. In this illustration, potential patients are admonished to follow "the sign" to the hospital, rather than attempting to obtain care at home. Judging from the clothing of those in the picture, it appears that the group being addressed is middle or upper class.

have the wards always full of visitors."[52] One private patient complained that she was required to wear "hospital garb," even though she had her own nightgowns. Even the private patient was subject to certain unattractive, if not humiliating, constraints: The hospital nightgown "was marked in big letters on the outside, with the words 'Private Patient Department,' to identify [her] probably if [she] got lost in the wards."[53]

The portrayal of the hospital as a hotel tended to undermine the authority and control exerted by the hospital staff. The warnings noted earlier against care for the patient by loved ones grew out of a belief in the hospital as a scientific, apersonal, and isolated environment. The home, by contrast, was characterized by personalized care provided by relatives, the family physician, and private-duty nurses. At St. Luke's Hospital, the superintendent discouraged friends and relatives from checking in with private patients because of the interference that such personalized and emotional concern could pose to hospital routine.[54]

Hospital patients in Brooklyn

As we have seen, the crisis in hospital finance promoted the acceptance of two important new features in the organization and support of large hospitals. First, it encouraged the gradual acceptance of the principle of patient payment as a significant mechanism of hospital support. Second, it made it necessary for hospitals to attract significant numbers of patients potentially capable of paying for the full cost of their care. To do this, hospitals added certain forms of class-distinct services that were unnecessary in the older working-class institutions. Large hospitals, particularly in Manhattan, constructed new wings and pavilions of private rooms and suites to attract private patients and served charity patients and those who could pay only in part in the old wards.

The smaller hospitals of Brooklyn faced significant problems in attempting to follow these models of hospital organization. As it turned out, the wealthy who were able to afford expensive private services frequently abandoned low-prestige Brooklyn institutions for the larger Manhattan facilities. The Brooklyn hospitals consequently found it difficult to attract the capital necessary for the construction of strictly isolated private wings. Furthermore, Brooklyn remained a "City of Homes" long after Manhattan became a city of apartment dwellers. Because they could easily be cared for in their homes, fewer Brooklyn patients needed the hospital.

Unable to fill their private rooms with wealthy private patients, small Brooklyn hospitals often sought payment from less wealthy blue-collar workers and petty clerks. Many institutions began to charge ward patients for services that were previously provided for minimal or no cost. In some cases, nonpaying working-class patients were actually denied access to independent hospital services. At Brooklyn Hospital, for instance, the trustees announced in 1900 that they were restricting the admission of free patients in an attempt to limit costs. "The Brooklyn Hospital trustees have decided to shut out part of the charity patients [in order to] keep expenses down," one journal noted. Accordingly, the census of free patients showed an immediate decline. From the beginning of the Depression in 1894 through 1900, the hospital census had shown a steady increase in the number of free patients admitted (see Figure 6). But the change in hospital policy quickly reversed this trend. In 1894, 997 free patients were admitted, and by 1900 this number had grown to 1,670. In 1901, however, the number of charity cases dropped by nearly 300 to 1,386. Not until 1913 would Brooklyn Hospital's census of free patients top the number attained in 1900.

The total number of hospital days used by free patients showed a similar trend (see Figures 7 and 8). These patients occupied the hospital for a total of 29,725 days in 1894, and by 1900, this figure grew to 34,014. The total number of free patient hospital days quickly plummeted, however, after the decision to limit access to free wards. Free patients occupied the hospital for only 25,512 days in 1900, and this figure would not again exceed 30,000 until 1914. The average hospital stay for a free patient declined significantly as well, dropping from 29.4 days in 1894 to 20.4 days per patient in 1900; by 1901, the average length of stay declined to 18.4 days.

The use of Brooklyn Hospital by paying and private-room patients showed the reverse tendency. The number of paying patients rose from 174 in 1892 to 381 in 1899, and 1900 saw the hospital census of paying patients rise even more dramatically to 609. It continued to rise slowly and unevenly until 1910. Although the number of charity patients stabilized between 1900 and 1910, the number of paying patients continued to rise (see Figure 6).

The percentage of patients who paid for part or all of their hospital care also rose after 1900. Between 1892 and 1899, the percentage of hospital patients who paid for their care had risen slowly from 14 to 19 percent. In 1900, however, the percentage of paying patients jumped significantly to almost 27 percent of the hospital's census. By 1901 over 35 percent of hospital patients paid for part or all of their care, and in 1902 over 43 percent of Brooklyn Hospital's patients were "pay patients." The paying patients accounted for about 40 percent of the

No. of patients

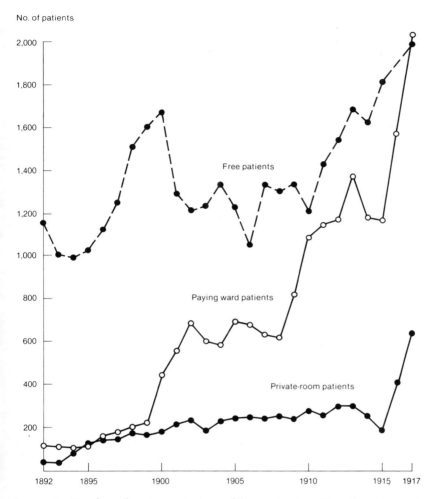

Figure 6. Number of paying, private, and free patients in Brooklyn Hospital, 1892–1917. (*Source*: Brooklyn Hospital, *Annual Reports*, 1892–1917.)

hospital's clients until 1910, when the figure jumped again to over 52 percent. The number of hospital days devoted to the use of paying patients also rose dramatically during the period. In 1892 paying patients used a total of only 4,212 hospital days (or 12.4 percent of all hospital days). By 1900 this figure had risen to 11,782 (or 25.7 percent), and by 1913 paying patients used 27,964 hospital days, or over 53 percent of the total.

No. of days of hospital care

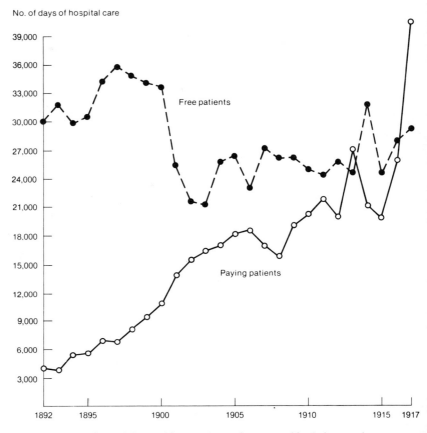

Figure 7. Number of days of hospital care by type of bed, free and paying, in Brooklyn Hospital, 1892–1917. (*Source*: Brooklyn Hospital, *Annual Reports*, 1892–1917.)

Brooklyn Hospital's growing dependence on paying patients is reflected in the percentage of its budget derived from this group. In 1892 only 12.2 percent of its costs came from hospital patients; by 1900 this figure had grown to 25.8 percent. Only five years later, in 1905, patient payments accounted for fully 61 percent of the hospital's income. By the end of the Progressive era, Brooklyn Hospital was no longer primarily a charity institution; substantial numbers of its clients paid for part or all of their care. The hospital, in effect, was dependent upon its patients as a primary source of income.[55]

The data provided in Figures 7 and 8 indicates interesting long-term changes in the payment of fees to the hospital. Whereas over 87 per-

No. of days of hospital care

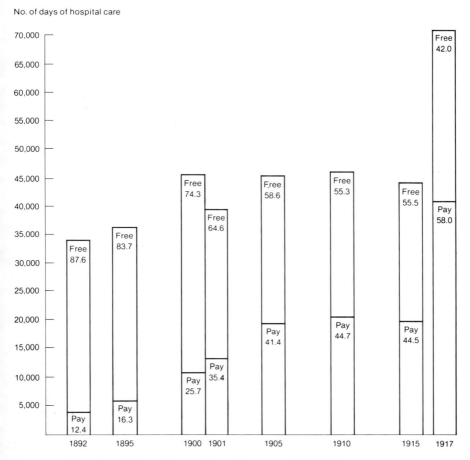

Figure 8. Number of days of hospital care by type of bed, with percentages of total, for Brooklyn Hospital, 1892–1917. (*Source*: Brooklyn Hospital, *Annual Reports*, 1892–1917.)

cent of all hospital days were used for the free patients in 1892, this figure steadily decreased during the period. Between 1900 and 1901, the number of days of free patient care dropped dramatically, by almost 9,000. Conversely, the hospital charged patients for services increasingly often, and there was a steady increase in the number of hospital days devoted to the care of paying patients. In 1900, 25.7 percent of all hospital days were used by such patients. Only a year after a change in the hospital's policy, however, over 35 percent of patients paid for their care.

The decision to cut out large numbers of formerly free patients had immediate effects on the number of services provided by the hospital. From 1892 until 1900, there had been a regular increase in the total number of days of hospital care provided by the hospital for its patients (Figure 8). In 1892 the hospital provided just over 34,000 days of hospital care to 1,323 patients. By 1900 the hospital provided nearly 46,000 days of hospital care to nearly 2,300 patients. In 1901, however, the slow but steady increase in hospital care was dramatically reversed. The number of days of hospital care provided dropped by over 6,000 to 39,510; furthermore, the fairly steady increase in the number of patients showed its first reverse in eight years, dropping to 2,149 (Figure 6). Steady growth in the number of patients treated at Brooklyn Hospital would not resume until 1909, when the patient load of the hospital increased to over 2,400.

It would be expected that, as hospitals changed from free services to services for which one paid, a greater percentage of patients would be from higher socio-economic groups. One might also expect that private rooms would be in high demand, and private nursing and other services widely used. In fact, private services were not very widely used, nor were wealthy patients flocking to the hospital. Only about 10 percent of patients used private rooms even at the peak of their popularity, between 1902 and 1912 (see Figure 6). The real growth in paying patient accommodations occurred in the number of persons using the pay *wards* of the hospital, not private rooms. These clients were distinguished from the charity patients by their ability to pay for part of their hospital care, and by their physical location in the hospital. Whereas only 10 percent of all hospital patients were paying patients throughout the 1890s, the number of paying ward patients began to increase dramatically in the early 1900s. In 1899 there were 228 paying ward patients at Brooklyn Hospital, representing just over 11 percent of all patients in the facility. In 1900, however, this number jumped to 439, or over 19 percent of all patients. By 1902, 679 patients, or 32 percent of all patients, were in paying wards. This percentage remained relatively stable until 1910, when it rose to over 42 (see Figure 6). It appears, then, that the growth in income from patients was not from the wealthier private-room patients, but from *paying ward* patients.

In addition, available data on the occupations of hospital patients confirms that the widening use of the paying wards occurred without a corresponding rapid rise in the social class of the hospital's patients. Applying Stephan Thernstrom's categories for the determination of occupational groups to patients in Brooklyn Hospital, I found the class makeup of patients for the years 1892 through 1904 (see Table 5). It appears that, between these years, there was a slow but steady rise in the social class of the patients, but this rise was slower than the corresponding rise in the use of paying services. In 1892, for instance, slightly less than 13 percent of all patients held white-collar jobs, whereas over 87 percent held blue-collar skilled or unskilled positions. By 1895 white-collar workers made up nearly 16 percent of the hospital patient population, and working-class patients about 84 percent. By 1900 white-collar workers accounted for almost 20 percent and blue-collar workers for just over 80 percent of the patient population.

Nearly all the growth in percentage of white-collar patients was in Group II, which largely represented the clerks, peddlers, typists, and small shopkeepers listed in the hospital census. Upper income patients in Group I never made up more than 2.2 percent of the hospital's patients. Furthermore, the decline in the percentage of working-class patients occurred primarily in Group V, or among the unskilled day laborers. Groups III and IV, skilled and unskilled laborers, constituted 19.8 and 30.0 percent, respectively, of all patients in 1892, and 18.9 and 31.0 percent of patients by 1904. Group V, however, the least-skilled members among blue-collar workers, found that Brooklyn Hospital's services were less and less available to them. In 1892 these workers made up fully 37 percent of the hospital's clients. By 1904 they composed less than 26 percent of the patient population. Presumably, these patients were now going to the city's growing municipal hospital system.

The proportion of white-collar workers using the hospital rose by about 12 percent between 1892 and 1904. The rise in the percentage of paying patients was considerably larger. This finding indicates that at least some working-class patients now were charged for services they previously received free. Between 1892 and 1904, the percentage of paying patients rose from just under 14 to just over 38, an increase of nearly 200 percent. Almost all paying patients in 1892 were in Groups I and II; by 1904, however, these groups could only account for fewer than two of every three patients who paid for all or part of their hospital services. If the bulk of white-collar workers paid at least some of the costs of their hospital stays in 1892, then nearly all the paying patients would be accounted for; if this was the case, few blue-collar workers were charged for hospital stays. By 1904, however, at least 14 percent of those paying for services were blue-collar workers, the group that, twelve years earlier, had received these services free of charge.

Far from becoming a middle-class institution, the hospital was still predominantly a working-class facility during the Progressive era.

Table 5. *Social class of patients in Brooklyn Hospital, 1892–1904*

	Occupational category[a]					Total	No occupation and house-keepers[b]
	I	II	III	IV	V		
1892							
No. of patients	6	116	188	285	354	949	360
% of total	0.63	12.22	19.81	30.03	37.19	100	
1893							
No. of patients	4	79	173	258	334	848	223
% of total	0.47	9.32	20.4	30.42	39.39	100	
1894							
No. of patients	8	112	174	257	434	985	210
% of total	0.81	11.37	17.66	26.09	44.06	100	
1895							
No. of patients	9	109	158	228	245	749	345
% of total	1.2	14.55	21.09	30.44	32.71	100	
1896							
No. of patients	6	140	184	262	250	842	442
% of total	0.71	16.63	21.85	31.12	29.69	100	
1897							
No. of patients	8	141	160	381	277	967	484
% of total	0.83	14.58	16.55	39.4	28.65	100	
1898							
No. of patients	10	218	458	555	351	1,592	189
% of total	0.63	13.69	28.77	34.86	22.05	100	

Year								
1899								
No. of patients	27	190	222	458	320	1,217	647	
% of total	2.22	15.61	18.24	37.63	26.29	100		
1900								
No. of patients	17	275	265	561	365	1,483	676	
% of total	1.15	18.54	17.87	37.83	24.61	100		
1901								
No. of patients	15	370	339	489	396	1,609	540	
% of total	0.93	23.0	21.07	30.39	24.61	100		
1902								
No. of patients	18	390	326	473	426	1,633	381	
% of total	1.1	23.88	19.96	28.96	26.09	100		
1903								
No. of patients	17	351	317	582	385	1,652	390	
% of total	1.03	21.25	19.19	35.23	23.31	100		
1904								
No. of patients	18	378	308	505	420	1,629	401	
% of total	1.1	23.2	18.91	31.0	25.78	100		

[a] For a full description of these categories, see Stephan Thernstrom, *The Other Bostonians: Poverty and Progress in the American Metropolis, 1880–1970* (Cambridge, Mass.: Harvard University Press, 1973).

[b] It is unclear whether "Housekeeper" refers to what we might consider a rooming-house manager, to a housewife, or to a servant. If a manager is meant, this might be judged a white-collar occupation. Servants or housewives could be considered blue-collar groups. Probably the "Housekeeper" category was primarily blue collar, in which case the hospital served an even larger proportion of blue-collar workers than these statistics indicate. Elimination of the category tends to mask the working-class nature of the hospital's clientele.

Source: Brooklyn Hospital, *Annual Reports*, 1892–1904.

What changed was that larger numbers of working-class persons paid for the hospital's services. Presumably, the group of laborers who were no longer admitted to independent hospitals were accommodated in the expanding public hospital system.

Information from other hospitals gives a slightly different cast to the general trend noted at Brooklyn Hospital. Using the information gathered by Thomas Kessner in his study of Jewish and Italian social mobility in Brooklyn and New York, it is possible to compare the occupational makeup of Brooklyn Hospital's patient population and Brooklyn's poor Italian and Jewish populations.[56] It becomes clear that the patients in Brooklyn Hospital were from a lower socioeconomic group than even the newest of immigrant groups in Brooklyn. In 1892, for instance, over 24 percent of Brooklyn's Russian Jewish households were in white-collar occupations, compared to less than 13 percent of Brooklyn Hospital's patients. In 1904 the percentage of patients with white-collar positions had surpassed 24, but 39 percent of Russian Jewish households had white-collar family heads. By the early 1900s the oldest hospital in Brooklyn still served a large portion of the city's working class, although unskilled laborers composed a smaller proportion of its patient population than in the past.[57]

Available birth certificates for the maternity wards of Brooklyn Hospital illustrate an interesting paradox that plagued those hospital administrators who expanded services in anticipation of large white-collar patient demand. Specifically, when new services were opened, the initial effect was to increase the percentage of blue-collar workers in the service. Brooklyn Hospital, for instance, opened its new Low Maternity service in 1894 and found that its service now attracted larger numbers of working-class, rather than white-collar, patients. In the years before 1895, when the building opened all of its new wards and rooms, 76.7 percent of the husbands of patients using the service held blue-collar occupations. Between 1895 and 1900, after the opening of the enlarged facility, the fathers of newborns were even more dramatically drawn from blue-collar occupations: At this point only 13 percent held white-collar jobs (see Table 6). As a number of hospital administrators pointed out, throughout the period the largest demand for services in hospitals still existed primarily among working-class groups.

Patient statistics from the Jewish Hospital of Brooklyn show that its largely Jewish patient population was very willing to utilize hospital services, irrespective of occupation. This hospital, located in the growing Russian Jewish neighborhood near Eastern Parkway, serviced large numbers of immigrants who were moving to Brooklyn from New York's lower East Side. A sample drawn from the patient records

Table 6. *Occupations of fathers of newborns at Brooklyn Hospital, 1892–1900*

	Occupational category[a]					
	I	II	III	IV	V	Total[a]
1892–1895						
No. of fathers	2	17	16	14	11	60
% of total	2.9	25	23.5	20.6	16.2	88.2
1896–1900						
No. of fathers	4	21	50	73	64	212
% of total	1.9	9.9	23.5	34.3	30	99.6

[a] For 1892–1895 not all birth certificates were noted for fathers' occupations. Mothers' occupations were not noted in either period; the hospital assumed that they were housewives or mothers.
Source: Brooklyn Hospital, birth certificates, 1892–1900. See Thernstrom, *The Other Bostonians,* for an elaboration of the categories used.

shows that the hospital, between 1907 (its first year of full service) and 1917, drew only about 60 to 80 percent of its patients from blue-collar occupations. The rest were primarily clerks and storekeepers.

Interestingly, it appears that admissions to the Jewish Hospital reflected almost exactly the occupational structure of Brooklyn's Russian Jewish community as a whole: About one-third of the community held white-collar positions and two-thirds, blue-collar jobs.[58] Russian Jews of all classes seem to have been willing to utilize the Jewish Hospital.[59]

At Methodist Hospital, low white-collar demand and large blue-collar need affected the makeup of patients in the hospital's wards and rooms (see Table 7). Throughout the 1890s there was a steady increase in the percentage of white-collar workers using the facility, but in the early 1900s, after the hospital expanded its service, this trend was reversed. The number of patients using the hospital in 1890 and 1895 remained relatively stable at about 500. By 1900, however, the patient census had reached 955, and by 1905 it was over 1,350.[60] Whereas over 27 percent of the hospital's patients were white-collar workers by 1895, however, less than 17 percent held white-collar jobs by 1905. As the hospital opened more beds, larger numbers of working-class patients sought its services, and the hospital administration, spurred by Bird S. Coler's new city ordinance guaranteeing municipal payment for working-class patients (see Chapter 5), quickly filled the new beds with city patients.

As institutions became increasingly tied to patient payments as an important source of funding, subtle and at times confusing patterns of payment and patient treatment developed. As Frank Tucker had

Table 7. *Patients at Methodist Hospital, 1890–1905*

	Occupational category							
	I	II	III	IV	V	Total[a]	White collar	Blue collar
1890								
No. of patients	9	74	94	164	149	490	83	407
% of total	1.84	15.1	19.18	33.47	30.41	100	16.94	83.06
1895								
No. of patients	21	120	122	171	85	519	141	378
% of total	4.05	23.12	23.51	32.95	16.38	100	27.17	72.83
1900								
No. of patients	23	230	211	233	258	955	253	702
% of total	2.41	24.08	22.09	24.4	27.02	100	26.49	73.51
1905								
No. of patients	35	183	122	260	723	1,323	218	1,105
% of total	2.65	13.83	9.22	19.65	54.65	100	16.48	83.52

[a] Totals do not include the categories "Housekeeper," "Student," "No Occupation," "Unknown," and "Scholar." For the "Housekeeper" category, see fn. *b* to Table 5, earlier in this chapter.
Source: Methodist Hospital, *Annual Reports,* 1890–1905. See Thernstrom, *The Other Bostonians,* for an elaboration of the categories used.

pointed out, services to the poor had to be decreased if room was to be made for the rich.[61] This was hardly an easy transformation for many institutions, however. The city's guarantee of payment for certain groups of poor persons and the idiosyncratic expansion of a number of facilities allowed at least temporarily for some expansion in certain services for working-class groups. But the long-term effect on hospital patients was truly severe: A rationalized, systematic separation of services, institutions, wards, and rooms was established. Patients came to accept services that the hospital deemed appropriate for their social class.

4   Conflict in the new hospital

Despite significant efforts to attract merchants and other white-collar workers by advertising comfortable accommodations and new services, hospital trustees were forced to admit that only a few more such patients actually came to the hospital. By and large the hospital was charging the very working-class patients who had previously used its services without charge, and these patients were bringing in only limited funds. Trustees came to realize that even if middle-class clients were influenced by pleasant accommodations and advertising, they were still the patients of private doctors and would enter the hospital only at those doctors' suggestion. Because family doctors would actually determine whether professionals, businessmen, and other people able to pay used the hospital, trustees came to see the necessity of forming an alliance with them.

For reasons related to their status in the hospital, even the most enthusiastic trustees could not help but have reservations about increasing the privileges of physicians. Throughout the nineteenth century, hospital trustees had direct control over the institutions they served, and their role was to function as the community's judge of who was worthy of admission to the facility. Once admitted, patients found that the trustees visited them regularly and took a personal, albeit paternalistic, interest in them. By the end of the century a number of things had caused control to begin slipping out of the trustees' hands. When hospital stays were shortened, trustees found it more difficult to oversee the physical and moral improvement of patients. Industrial accidents, the lack of doctors' services in poorer neighborhoods, and the growth in patient demand for basic health care shifted the locus of admissions to the dispensary and the emergency room. Consequently, the physicians who staffed these services became increasingly important in admissions decisions once made by the trustees. At the same time hospital and dispensary administrators, faced with an increasingly complex hospital, began to make decisions without consulting trustees.

94

Opening the hospital: the question of increased staff privileges for doctors

The battle over increasing the number of physicians on staff was fought in many hospital boardrooms among trustees already feeling a loss of control. To help calm the initial fears of trustees, suggestions for staff enlargement generally contained a clause making it clear that the participation of doctors in the hospital would be very limited. In 1894, for instance, George White, a trustee at Brooklyn Hospital, called the attention of the board to the many vacant rooms for private patients and urged that some action be taken whereby "physicians of standing would have the use of these rooms for their patients without the responsibility attaching to the Hospital."[1] The board intended to increase the number of physicians associated with the hospital, but to keep those physicians and their patients isolated from the staff physicians and charity patients. In this way trustees hoped to maintain their traditional role as guardians of the charity hospital and to protect their institution from large numbers of private doctors, whom the trustees often considered unschooled and uncouth.

The struggle over enlarging the staff at Brooklyn Hospital continued from around 1894 to 1901. In fact, every trustee meeting in the beginning of 1901 was the scene of a debate over staff enlargement. "Though the Committee has given the subject the most careful consideration, no satisfactory method of decreasing the expenses or of increasing the income has been discovered, though the necessity for some prompt action is fully recognized," noted the report of the board's special committee on the financial crisis of the hospital. "The recommendation . . . that the private accommodations of the Hospital be increased and thrown open to the regular profession of the City is reluctantly though unanimously endorsed by the Committee, who recognize . . . the numerous objections to such a course." The committee felt obliged to accept the plan because "no better suggestion [for increasing income] has been made."[2]

In addition to the introduction of local physicians and their patients into the hospital, the plan called for the further curtailment of charity services by de facto conversion of charity wards into paying wards when demand from private patients justified the change. It was "resolved, that the private accommodations of the Hospital be increased by converting Wards 10, 11, 12, and 13 or so much thereof as may be necessary, into Pay Wards without material alterations or expense, and that the private accommodations of the Hospital be thrown open to the regular profession of the City."[3] Those members disturbed by this move sought to delay the introduction of large numbers of private

HOSPITAL MANAGEMENT

February, 1918
Vol. V, No. 1

608 S. Dearborn
Street,
Chicago

Published in the Interest of Executives in Every Department of Hospital Work
Entered as second class matter May 14, 1917, at the post office at Chicago, Ill., under the act of March 3, 1879.

Get Together and Your Problems Will Disappear

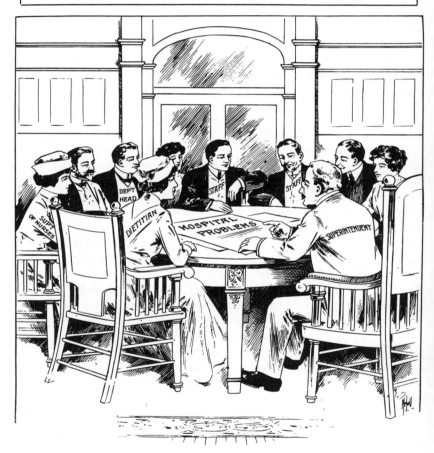

By the end of the Progressive era, what had been a relatively simple labor–
management organization at the turn of the century was becoming increasingly complicated and fragmented. In these three comments on the growing
complexities, *Hospital Management* suggests that the situation will improve only
if the various groups of workers coordinate their efforts and only if manage-

96

HOSPITAL
MANAGEMENT

Published in the Interest of Executives in Every Department of Hospital Work

Will It Come to This?

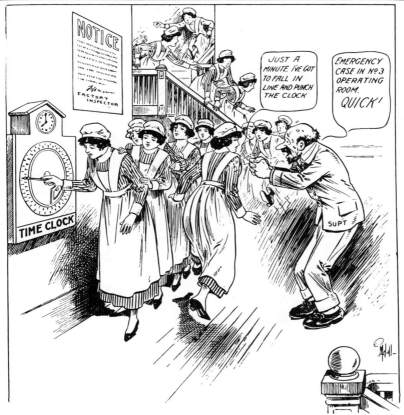

News Item—Women's labor laws regulating the hours of hospital nurses are so severe that many institutions are putting in time-clocks, to make sure that their students will not "work over-time."

ment adopts new "scientific" work-saving devices to cut down on the hospital's dependence on human labor. Developing new "factorylike" practices, however, had special drawbacks for an institution that was highly labor-intensive, as the illustration of nurses at the time clock points out.

97

HOSPITAL
MANAGEMENT

November, 1918
Vol. VI, No. 4

417 S. Dearborn Street, Chicago

Published in the Interest of Executives in Every Department of Hospital Work

The Labor-Saver Makes a Popular Employe

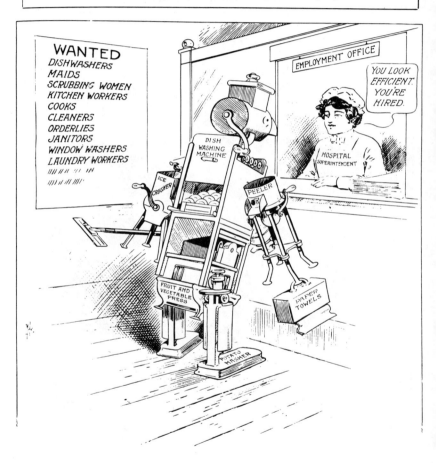

community physicians,[4] but by 1903 the opposition on the board to expanded visiting privileges for community physicians was overcome.

In quick succession the board adopted a number of measures that extended physicians' access to private services. In February 1903 "privileges of the private rooms and private wards" were extended "to the Dispensary Staff, the clinical assistants" and the anesthetist.[5] In March the board agreed on the appointment of an auxiliary staff of ten new physicians, "who shall have the privilege of the private rooms and operating rooms."[6] By December, the trustees began drawing up "rules governing the Visiting Staff in the matter of their fees."[7]

A similar decision was impending at New York Hospital around this time. Superintendent George Ludlam noted that as "far as [he could] ascertain, the patronage of the private rooms in hospitals is dependent very largely upon the interest and active cooperation of the Medical Staff." He pointedly told his board of governors that "most of the private patients are sent by the professional gentlemen who are attending them," and because the private rooms and services were still largely empty, it was therefore necessary "to consider the question of extending the [hospital] privilege more widely." The same week, another of New York Hospital's spokesmen, Howard Townsend, called the board's attention to the fact that Roosevelt Hospital had just recently "decided to extend the privilege of the Private Patient Pavilion" to new physicians who might bring their patients with them. To Townsend, it was "very clear . . . that some such step should be taken."[8]

Once trustees on a hospital board decided to enlarge the staff, they had no trouble attracting physicians to the hospital. For a number of reasons, doctors had become increasingly interested in the hospital by the early years of the new century. The growth of a belief in scientific medicine made doctors, particularly specialists and educators, eager for experience with new techniques and technologies. In the hospital's clinics, emergency rooms, and wards, doctors could gain experience with a wider variety of patients than could be found in private family practice. Certain illnesses rarely seen in individual practice were more likely to appear in the hospital. Hospitals also had the promise of available operating theaters, X-ray machines, autoclaves, and other expensive equipment not justifiably purchased for the private office. In Manhattan, where there were a large number of medical schools, specialists and physicians in training actually competed for hospital appointments in order to gain clinical experience.[9]

It is important to understand that the development of new scientific techniques caused doctors to view themselves much more as scientists than they had previously. Increasingly, a doctor was considered competent only insofar as he had adequate clinical training and familiarity with techniques and procedures best learned in a hospital setting. For much of the nineteenth century, medical education had been largely an informal affair. Physicians were trained through apprenticeship or in schools of varying caliber with no uniform standards or requirements. Proprietary educational institutions provided little more than a few months of lectures and no clinical experience, and even more reputable institutions rarely provided their students with substantial exposure to hospital or clinic patients. By the end of the century, however, both proprietary and university-affiliated medical schools began to develop new curricula and standards in order to graduate students with minimal technical and diagnostic skills; and to meet these new requirements students sought hospital appointments.

The experience of Long Island College Hospital (LICH), a proprietary medical school in Brooklyn, illustrates the effect of rapidly changing scientific expectations on the standards of medical educators and institutions at the end of the century. Early in 1900, a doctor from Irondale, Ohio, wrote to Dr. Joseph Raymond, the secretary of the LICH faculty, to inquire about the possibilities of attaining a medical degree from the college. "I being a legal Registered Physician in the State of Ohio it is not compulsory for me to graduate [from a medical school]," he explained. "But [I] would like to be Recognized By Some Good Medical College and it would be impossible for me to leave my practice to attend a full term of lectures." He stated unabashedly that he would like to pay his tuition and "come and fetch my credentials and the affidavits of some . . . M.D. in regard to my ability [and] Reputation as a Physician and Surgeon." He thought that an M.D. degree from LICH would give him a competitive advantage over those doctors in the area who held diplomas from less prestigious western schools. Because he already had a state license, he too could "fetch" a diploma from a local medical school, he said, but he did "not want them [sic] as [he] had these graduates all around" him.[10] This physician wrote to LICH specifically because the school was on the East Coast, reputable, and a proprietary institution. His letter reflected a commonly held opinion that the significance of the M.D. degree added more to the status and social position of the practitioner than to any practical skills.

To his surprise, the physician was informed by Raymond that to receive an M.D. degree from LICH he would have to attend classes and complete a course of study that included a hospital rotation. The payment of a fee alone was not adequate for the degree. Under pressure from state licensing boards, medical schools like LICH had begun to demand rigorous training. In the 1890s the newly organized Association of American Medical Colleges began to develop minimal standards for medical education and promoted a three-year curriculum. In New York State, the Board of Medical Examiners forced schools to devote the first two years of their curriculum exclusively to demonstrations and lectures in the basic sciences and to laboratory work; the third year was for clinical work in a hospital or outpatient clinic.[11]

For many, particularly those trained in a previous era, these new standards and criteria for medical education were extremely disruptive. In May 1899, for instance, Henry Sanford, an important administrator in New York State's Department of Public Instruction, also began to correspond with Raymond. Sanford, whose son had not been graduated by the college, hoped to convince Raymond to reconsider his son's work and allow him to graduate. "I have heard with surprise and pain that my son, James, has not been passed for graduation," he wrote. "This seems very strange for although you have written me . . . during the past two years in regard to the payments of tuition and other dues, you have never once intimated that he was not doing good work." Sanford judged that the payment of tuition to this proprietary medical school constituted a contract between him and the institution. After all, his son had transferred to LICH from the older, more prestigious Columbia College of Physicians and Surgeons in New York only two years earlier for the expressed purpose of attaining a degree on time: "You, of course, fully understood that when he transferred to [LICH] . . . it was for the purpose of completing the course at this time."[12] After a series of angry letters in which Sanford threatened to use his power in the state against the school, he was forced to acknowledge that his son would not graduate. It appeared that James had failed no fewer than six subjects.[13]

For practitioners working in communities where scientific medicine was not as central, and clinical experience not as important, other factors made the hospital appointment attractive. In Brooklyn, for instance, where there was only one medical school, a hospital appointment signified acceptance by the community's moral leaders and social elites, and consequently conferred a fair amount of social and professional status. In communities where the medical profession was severely overcrowded, a hospital appointment had the advantage of providing practitioners with access to new patients, whom they could charge or take with them into private practice. It is ironic that hospital trustees welcomed family practitioners to the hospital precisely because they hoped these practitioners would bring their private patients, whereas the private doctors sought out the hospital because they needed patients and hoped the hospital would provide them.

As more physicians were admitted to hospital staffs, those who were excluded became resentful. Some family practitioners who were unable to gain appointments to the hospital saw those with appointments as little other than thieves plotting to take patients away from them. Far removed from the increasing sophistication of the developing specialties, many community doctors saw little of value in hospital care other than the competitive advantage it provided in a highly crowded field. "Why is it that when our patients enter a hospital we must surrender them to self-styled and Lord-knows how appointed professors (?) who assume ownership and charge of them . . . in absolute disregard of our rights in the matter?" complained Lester D. Volk, a family practitioner who edited the *Medical Economist*, a journal devoted to protecting the struggling private practitioner. "If the patient . . . has money, then the great system of our modern hospital comes into play . . . The X-Ray man, pathologist and specialogist [*sic*], the attending and assistant – all exact their fees – but so far as the family doctor is concerned, the patient might just as well be a stranger in a strange land."[14] Private practitioners who resented the advantage the hospital provided some doctors called on trustees to "OPEN THE DOORS OF THE HOSPITALS TO THE MEDICAL PROFESSION,"[15] that is, to the entire medical profession. "The general practitioners, in large cities especially," felt that hospitals allowed their patients to drift into the hands of other doctors, "not infrequently an active competitor" of the referring physician.[16]

The fact was that hospitals were opening their doors to family doctors, although too slowly to satisfy them. As trustees were forced to search for paying patients, they found that very few practitioners had lucrative practices and those who did were often already associated with one or more institutions. As a result, hospitals often enlarged their staffs with local practitioners who had marginally successful practices and who could be counted on for only a few referrals a year. Often these practitioners were interested in attaining a hospital appointment more to draw on new patients and interesting cases than to serve the goals of the charity hospital. Bringing to the hospital their assumptions about good private practice, these community physicians were not used to or interested in the methods of practice required for efficiency and control in an institution.

Once hospital trustees began to admit more doctors to use of the hospital it became difficult for them to limit the number. "From the standpoint of the managers of a present-day American hospital," noted Lewis Stephen Pilcher in the *Long Island Medical Journal*, "the larger the number of physicians that can be crowded upon the staff of the insti-

Table 8. *Hospital affiliation among Brooklyn practitioners, 1890-1918*

	1890	1900	1910	1918	Total
No. of physicians with hospital affiliation	34	20	74	97	225
% of total for year	23.9	15.6	42.3	45.5	
No. of physicians without hospital affiliation	108	108	101	116	433
% of total for year	76.1	84.4	57.7	54.5	
Total	142	128	175	213	658

Note: $\chi^2 = 46.0$ with 3 *df*, sig. $> .005$.
Source: Sample drawn from *Medical Directories*, 1890, 1900, 1910, 1918.

tution the better, for each additional one means an additional coterie of possible supporters."[17] In Brooklyn it was certainly held that the larger the staff of physicians, the better. Between 1900 and 1910, for instance, the figure for hospital-affiliated physicians rose from 15.6 percent of Brooklyn's practitioners to over 42 percent (see Table 8). Many of the city's general and specialty facilities saw a rapid growth in the size of their staffs. Brooklyn Hospital expanded its visiting staff from 11 in 1890 to 57 in 1914. At Methodist Hospital the affiliated staff increased from 16 visiting and staff physicians in 1890 to 54 in 1914 (see Figure 9).

Overall, private physicians did bring in paying patients.[18] Abraham Abraham stated the position of many hospital trustees when he said in the Jewish Hospital's *Annual Report* of 1903, "Your Board has the assurance of the most prominent surgeons and physicians of this borough that we can fill the entire building, if we so desire, with patients who are willing to pay liberally for superior accommodations."[19] For this reason trustees were generally happy about the inclusion of more physicians on the hospital staff. But they were less pleased about the potentially profound influence of this change on their ability to control the staff. Trustees first sought out those practitioners who had been trained in the hospital and who were likely to be loyal to the hospitals' traditions. The superintendent at New York Hospital pointed out that there were "three classes [of practitioners] which might be considered as eligible" for hospital appointments. The first group was "the staff of the Out-Patient Department," and the second was "former members of the House Staff now practicing in the city" – all of whom were aware of the hospital's organization and purpose. The members of the third group were "reputable practitioners in the city not connected with

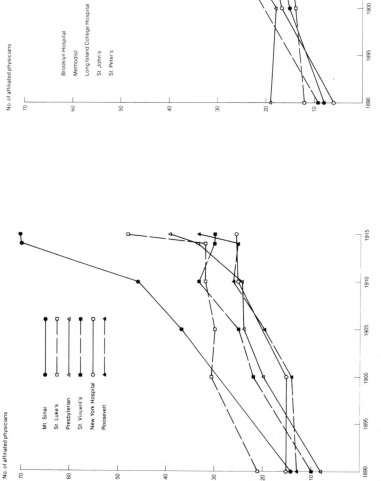

Figure 9. Number of hospital-affiliated physicians in specified (*left*) Manhattan and (*right*) Brooklyn hospitals, 1890–1915. (*Source: Medical Registers and Medical Directories, 1890, 1900, 1905, 1910, 1914, 1915.*)

the Hospital." Introducing this last group, he explained, "would be a radical departure from long established order, and, probably, would not meet with favor." Although the superintendent himself seemed interested in these practitioners, because their counterparts had been used by "hospitals in other cities," he recognized that there were serious issues regarding their ultimate loyalty to the institution and to the board of governors itself.[20]

The trustees' eagerness to admit "cooperative" doctors reflected their sense that the doctors posed a real threat to their power. Trustees realized that doctors had access to new medical procedures and techniques, that the doctors' authority in regard to these innovations was unquestionable, and that it was only a matter of time before they would test the strength of this newfound authority. Furthermore, because the number of doctors with hospital appointments had increased tremendously, the sheer force of their numbers would soon give them a kind of advantage over the trustees and administrators.

Trustees, physicians, and power

As the number of physicians affiliated with the hospital rose, doctors did begin to realize their potential for power in the hospital. Generally they first attempted to exert their authority over trivial issues, and they quickly met firm opposition from the trustees. At Brooklyn's Eastern District Hospital, for instance, the trustees accepted the resignations of three members of the medical staff rather than acquiesce to their request for a change in their daily fare of fishball soup. "The status of the fishball as an article of diet suitable for hard working physicians and surgeons is likely to be established in Williamsburg," the *New York Times* reported in October 1896. The doctors all objected to the daily diet of stewed prunes, the fishball, and "papier mâché rice pudding" and demanded instead "steak two or three times a week for dinner, roast beef twice, clam chowder once, and oysters once." The superintendent, faced by a board of trustees seeking to limit costs, accepted the resignations and stated that "the fare was as good as could be afforded with the sum at his disposal."[21]

The feud over fishballs reflected a battle that had been raging at the hospital for at least the previous ten months. A small institution in the Williamsburg section of Brooklyn, the hospital had been struggling through the financial depression and had been faced with a shrinking budget. In March 1896 the hospital's trustees had dismissed the entire medical staff, claiming that the "old staff was dropped" in order to "centralize responsibility" at the facility. This act indicated that the

Eastern District Hospital trustees still considered that they maintained ultimate authority within the institution. The doctors were "quite angry over what they term the indignity implied by the sudden dismissal," but they lodged no effective complaint.[22]

Other small institutions also found trustees and doctors at odds over a range of seemingly trivial matters. In 1894 ten physicians at the Eastern District Homeopathic Hospital tendered their resignation after two years of quarrels with the board. The ostensible issue was "an order prohibiting the physicians playing cards and other games in the hospital." The climax was reached when the trustees asked the doctors to sign "a circular dedicating themselves to the welfare of the hospital." This circular reminded the doctors that their appointments were tentative and called upon them to subordinate themselves to the authority of the trustees, in a manner reminiscent of an earlier era of trustee-physician relations. "In the event of my reappointment I agree to conform to the rules and regulations by your Board," it began. The statement then called upon doctors to attend to their clinic, ward, and other professional duties. "The doctors indignantly refused to sign the circular and decided that it was time for them to sever their connection with the institution," reported the *Times*. After a conference with the board president, at which time he "refused to recall the offensive circular," the doctors resigned.[23]

Whereas the Williamsburg hospital battles dealt with relatively trivial issues like food and games, other hospitals saw more serious threats to board authority during the 1890s. In some cases doctors went on strike to protest working conditions or the structure of relationships in the hospital. Generally trustees were not hesitant to fire physicians. At Brooklyn's largest institution, St. John's Episcopal Hospital, the authority of the nurses was significant enough to undermine the position of the young physicians, and three interns were asked to resign when they took issue with the actions of one of the nurses. "An examination was held," reported the *Tribune*, and the board "made clear to Dr. Curry that his relations with the hospital were somewhat inharmonious." The hospital's superintendent, Reverend A. C. Bunn, added that the "work of the hospital had not been impaired in the slightest degree by the withdrawal of the three physicians."[24]

At another, smaller Brooklyn facility, German Hospital, conflict between the head nurse and the medical staff led to the resignations of a number of doctors. The physicians "requested the Board of Trustees to ask for the resignation of Miss Ella D. Kurtz, the head nurse, charging her with interfering in matters not under her supervision," reported the *Tribune* in 1906. Rather than reprimand the nurse, however, the trustees reprimanded the physicians for their attempt to "run the whole hospital."[25]

Although trustees were able to use their traditional position of power to oppose the doctors for a while, ultimately they were dependent on doctors for their access to paying patients and for their medical expertise and judgment. As medical information increased, specialists and other doctors made decisions on medical grounds that were outside the expertise of the lay trustee and superintendent. In 1893, for instance, "rumors reflecting upon the care exercised in some of the major operations performed in the hospital" came to the attention of trustees at Brooklyn Hospital. The trustees, unable to judge for themselves, asked a committee of physicians to evaluate the complaints. Not surprisingly, the physicians unanimously agreed that "the operations . . . were performed with care and every precaution."[26] The lay trustees had no recourse but to depend upon the professional integrity and judgment of their staff.

Two years later, however, the hospital's trustees noted that "rumors have reached the ears of individual members of this Board reflecting on the careful treatment of patients." Again, the physicians on the staff reported that the allegations were "utterly without foundations," and the trustees again accepted this position with no comment.[27] Frustrated by their inability to evaluate complaints, the trustees made a last attempt to exert their authority by passing a resolution to control the spread of rumors and negative criticism. At their March 1895 meeting they resolved "that all criticism of the staff or comments reflecting the management of this institution by anyone in the Service of the Hospital is absolutely forbidden." Furthermore, such criticism could "render the party implicated liable to immediate dismissal."[28]

The challenge posed by the doctors to the authority of the trustees was previously unheard of. For decades trustees had run their hospitals like large, patriarchal families. At their monthly meetings, they had made mundane administrative decisions as well as long-term policy decisions. They had decided on the amount and quality of the food and which patients to admit; they had hired medical and other staff members and planned renovations, construction, and fund raising. Usually their decisions had been enforced by the nonmedical superintendent and the head of nursing services, who, because they were often the only two full-time staff members hired by the trustees, oversaw the daily operations in the hospital. Superintendents were generally drawn from upper-middle-class groups or the clergy and nurses from the families of white-collar workers. As the only middle-class persons on the staff, the people in these positions were generally allowed a certain degree of autonomy over the working-class patients in the hospital. The few local doctors who functioned a few hours a week as attending physicians were subject to the control of upper-class trustees.[29] Most medical care was provided by interns or "house" staff, who were appointed for a year and who lived in the hospital, subject to the authority of the head nurse and superintendent. It was nearly inconceivable to trustees at that time that doctors might exert their authority in any significant way in the hospital.

Private patients and physicians' payments

Trustees who admitted doctors to the hospital in the hopes of drawing paying patients had no idea how complex the issue of payment would become. Private practitioners always had a more entrepreneurial relationship with their patients than did hospitals. Entirely dependent upon remunerations from the patients they treated in their homes and offices, private doctors were careful to foster the kind of personal relationships that would ensure the patient's patronage. When these private doctors became affiliated with hospitals, they brought with them the private model of practice. Trustees who saw the hospital as a place to care for many indigent patients had little patience for the kind of personalized care the physicians tried to deliver. Nor could the trustees have understood the physicians' need to "court" patients in order to justify billing them, because it never occurred to these financially pressed trustees that physicians would send patients their own bills.

Trustees eventually realized that doctors would charge their private patients, but they maintained that direct payment to private physicians should not be expected of patients in the whole institution. When physicians sought to extract fees from paying ward patients, they were opposed by administrators still committed to the notion of the hospital as charity. Ward patients were not required to pay for physician service, but only for hospital accommodations, and when they did pay for the physician, the administrator and not the doctor was to determine the amount.[30]

Physicians were quick to attack the protectionist attitude of many trustees. In 1906 the doctors at Methodist Hospital sent a letter to the trustees demanding that the older rules concerning the collection of fees be reviewed. The doctors objected that the concentration of power in the hands of lay administrators often debarred the physicians "from the privilege of collecting fees from patients they send to the wards who pay the regular ward rates." They argued that the distinction between the private patient in the private room and the paying patient in the hospital's ward was old-fashioned and prevented them from obtaining income. They obviously disagreed with the trustees' and superintendent's view "that no fee should be collected from any patient paying full ward rates who was unable to pay a physician's fee," because this view prevented them from working out their own financial arrangements with ward patients. From the perspective of private practitioners, the hospital administrator had redefined the old charity patients and now considered them "paying ward" patients. Why then could doctors not also consider them paying patients and determine their own fees? The administration maintained that it was up to the business office "to discover the exact financial ability of patients."[31]

As discussed earlier, many institutions had shifted from charity to paying service primarily at the expense of working-class patients who were now required to pay for services they had once received without charge. Although these people were now categorized as paying patients, trustees and administrators often maintained their paternalistic, protective attitude toward them. Recognizing that little more than their categorization had changed, superintendents tried to protect them from the imposition of fees by practitioners seeking to maximize their experience and their income. The hospital business office engaged in "a voluminous correspondence . . . to discover the exact financial ability of patients, so that no injustice shall be done the Hospital, the patients, or the Physicians."[32]

Doctors objected that the private rooms for which they were allowed to make separate arrangements with patients were largely underutilized and often vacant. As late as 1908, the superintendent reported that "from six to a dozen [private room] beds were always vacant, and for several months in the year nearly half of the beds" were empty.[33] An executive committee report in the same year revealed that a "careful study of our increased private facilities and the number of patients cared for, reveals the fact that our facilities are greater than the demands of our Staff upon them."[34] The medical staff, unable to supply sufficient private patients, needed access to large numbers of ward patients in order to assure themselves of adequate experience and recompense. In such a situation, conflict over control of those paying ward patients was inevitable.

Doctors saw the difficulty of convincing patients to pay them. Heber Hoople, a vocal Brooklyn physician who joined the staff of the Williamsburg Hospital, recognized the need to alter the attitudes of patients if physicians were to count on fees from them. Hospitals, he noted, were "supported by charity, donations, grants, etc., and therefore the presumption is, at least as far as the public wards are concerned, that all treatment is to be free." Hoople noted that "the right to pay depending on the ability to pay, is not recognized in law [and] if patients have to pay, then [the hospital] is not a public institution." Remarking on a Toronto lawsuit in which a judge ruled that a physician working in a charity institution had no right to charge a fee to his patients, Hoople recommended that the profession demand "nothing less than . . . a readjustment of [the hospital's] foundation." In the first place, "if the only service to be rendered within it must be free, then [the] patient able to pay [has] no right there and should [be] as rigidly excluded as the poor patient [is] made welcome." Hoople recommended that a physician provide only as much service as he is paid for and that he "only serve well one who is able to pay well": All the "sentimental nonsense about the inhumanity of it to the contrary," archaic, unbusinesslike attitudes, even in the context of charity, served only as a "cloak [that] covers too many unpaid doctor's bills."[35] Hoople's attitude reflected the general feeling of private physicians working in the hospital that gratuitous hospital care, based upon the paternalism of an earlier era, was outmoded in a business-oriented society.

When doctors encountered opposition from trustees, they sometimes sought legal help in maintaining their right to charge hospital patients for professional services. In May 1902 Gordon R. Fowler, a surgeon affiliated with the Brooklyn, Methodist, and German hospitals, sued eight patients who had refused or hesitated to pay for his professional services. "This is a fight for the sake of a principle," Fowler explained. He asserted that both hospitals and "surgeons have suffered . . . a long time and I propose to see whether or not the law will allow us to be cheated out of what is due us."[36] Fowler was "determined to try out in the courts the question of whether or not a man with plenty of money could go into a public hospital and get the benefits of a skillful and high-priced operation for nothing." When one of the defendants offered to settle out of court, Fowler declined to settle, again "saying that he didn't care so much for the money as for the principle."[37] "These suits are test cases," he insisted, "and by them I hope to vindicate a principle that is being abused in every hospital."[38]

Doctors intended to charge not only clients who could obviously afford their services, but also those indigent and working-class patients for whom the hospital had always been free. "For years certain persons have imposed upon physicians and hospitals by claiming that they were too poor to pay for dangerous and skillful operations," Fowler claimed. "I immediately made up my mind that my professional services and skill were worth something and I brought suit against [some of these people] . . . It is about time that the medical profession put a stop to these impositions."[39]

Fowler also sought to establish the legal right of surgeons and physicians to collect professional fees exclusive of the hospital's charge. When minimal charges to ward patients were instituted on a widespread basis, many patients assumed that the hospital bill included professional services. This meant that, except for the salaried house physicians who received a minimal subsidy including food and shelter, physicians were receiving no financial remuneration directly from the hospital. "Judge Van Wart . . . holds that patients who accept the services of physicians and surgeons in hospitals must pay for such services, even though there has been no agreement on the part of the patient to do so," reported the *Eagle*. "It was charged that patients go [to the German Hospital] and pay for board and nursing at the rate of the hospital, $7 per week, and accept the treatment of the surgeons and physicians there and refuse to pay."[40]

From the patients' point of view, however, hospitals were responsible for providing all associated services, including physicians' care: "The money they paid the hospital," according to the *Eagle's* report of their claim, "covered all treatment by the physicians and surgeons connected therewith." Another of Fowler's patients at Methodist Hospital repeated this defense, but to no avail. "It is not disputed that the defendant paid the sums of money . . . but there is a dispute as to what the money was paid for." Fowler maintained that the money was paid for board and nursing services, not physicians' services.[41]

The fight to establish the right of physicians to provide separate bills for their services indicates an interesting point about the nineteenth-century hospital. As has been pointed out, physicians at that time constituted a very small and insubstantial portion of a hospital's staff and played a much less significant role in the hospital than is the case today.[42] The hospital of the era, a place of moral reform as well as medical care, saw medical services as only *one* of the institution's many functions. When patients began receiving separate bills from the hospital and from their physicians, it was clear that the status of the doctor had increased significantly and that doctors saw themselves as outside the hospital structure. Furthermore, when hospitals were solely charities and trustees made no attempt to charge patients, doctors had made no move to collect fees. Only as doctors began to perceive a change in the overall orientation of the hospital did they begin to object to working without pay.

Organizational battles

Trustees and superintendents, reeling from the newly attained authority of physicians within their institutions, sought at least to limit the organizational control that private physicians could assert. In the prewar days of the summer of 1914, the superintendent of Methodist Hospital wrote a long memo to the hospital's lay executive committee of the board of managers outlining his position on a number of hospital issues, including the seemingly trivial matter of noise in the halls. It appears that the wards and halls of the hospital resounded with the clatter of the buzzers, bells, and whistles that were employed to call specific practitioners to attend their patients in a private room or ward. For Superintendent Kavanagh, the "infamous whistle," the ancestor of the "beeper," was a concrete manifestation of the complexity and confusion the introduction of private doctors had brought to the hospital. "It is one thing to conduct a hospital with hundreds of patients when they are all cared for in great wards by a few physicians who have no private practice," the superintendent observed. "It is another thing to care for hundreds of patients where a large percentage are private patients, and a dozen doctors may be treating them, and each doctor is anxious to stand in well with the patient, and friends of the patient, and not always particularly friendly to the hospital which is serving them."[43] To stand in well with their patients the doctors demanded new services for them – private rooms for those unwilling to enter the hospital's wards, private nursing, better-quality food, and more flexible visiting hours.

Methodist's Superintendent Kavanagh continued to wish for the days when the hospital had been a simple enough organization to permit him to solve problems like noise in the hall by issuing a direct order: "I should get rid of the whistle in six weeks if I could reorganize the Hospital and run it on a plan as simply as Kings County." In Kavanagh's view, the absence of private practice physicians at Kings County Hospital allowed its superintendent simply to summon any house physician when a patient needed care. Under such a system, there would be no need for the complicated buzzer system that characterized Methodist Hospital. "In our effort . . . to please our Attendings," he observed, "we have built up an intricate piece of machinery, which is becoming more and more difficult to handle every day." Far from being a quiet refuge in which the patient could escape the pressure of the outside world, the new Methodist Hospital was becoming a busy machine shop. Kavanagh quoted a visitor to the hospital who had sat in a hall for an hour and "was amazed at what [he] saw." He "had seldom been in a place where so much was going on. The nurses and orderlies on the floor; the attendings arriving, the friends of patients coming, messenger boys with flowers . . ."[44]

Kavanagh noted that the introduction of large numbers of practitioners had created other more profound changes. The loyalty of physicians to their private patients often created differences of opinion between the superintendent and the attending staff. Doctors, viewing the hospital as an adjunct of their private service, used it as a personal workshop complete with the advantages of nursing, surgical, medical, and ancillary backup services. They insisted on providing the kind of individualized care characteristic of their private practice rather than the more impersonal, ward-based care necessary for the smooth running of the hospital. Doctors also tended to disassociate themselves from responsibility for the hospital's policy at the very time when hospital policy was seeking to adjust itself to the wishes of the private doctors upon whom the facility depended for patients.

Kavanagh noted the paradoxical position in which the doctors put the hospital. They pressed hospital administrators to accept private patients at the practitioners' and patients' convenience and then criticized the administrators if the accommodations provided were not ideal. "Certain of our doctors try to force us to receive patients for which we have no accommodations," Kavanagh complained. "They are indifferent as to where we place them so long as they can get them in. Then the friends of the patients complain and, as a rule, the doctor does not try to shield us by explaining our difficulties." Kavanagh felt "that some of our doctors rejoice more in criticism made concerning the Hospital than in its praise."[45]

Kavanagh was correct in his perception that the hospital was dealing with doctors who had different interests from those of physicians previously associated with their institutions. From a small group of practitioners who depended upon hospital trustees for their appointments and positions, doctors had grown into a substantial segment of the hospital staff upon whom the trustees depended for paying patients and for the provision of medical care. Because doctors were the group singularly responsible for pleasing paying patients, they became all the more essential to the facility. The trustees were faced with a dilemma: Insofar as they satisfied the doctors' educational and financial needs, they contributed to the demise of the charity hospital. Although the superintendent of Methodist could declare that "the man who fails as a teamworker in the Hospital fails in every way,"[46] it was clear that the collective interest in charity work was giving way to a new entrepreneurial and individualistic form of health care delivery.

The competitive, entrepreneurial interests of the physicians eventually led them into conflicts with each other that disrupted the hospital even more severely. Early in the century doctors sought hospital appointments to gain experience in a specialty or surgical setting, as well as to gain access to patients for their private practices. In their attempts to maximize the number of patients under their own sponsorship, doctors soon found that practitioners with more rank and position in the hospital were controlling the most interesting patients.[47] At Methodist Hospital, the house staff of young, newly graduated doctors often found themselves unable to receive proper clinical experience because large numbers of older attending physicians and their assistants controlled and usurped hospital privileges for themselves.

By 1910 Methodist Hospital's "House Staff was in a state of rebellion." House physicians and surgeons resigned their posts to protest the control the attending physicians exerted over such things as access to hospital beds, the use of the operating room, and consultations in interesting cases. The house staff "charged that the surgeons did not give them a fair opportunity to see, and to learn; that in almost every case in the Operating Room, the Attending used as his first assistant his own personal assistant . . . and that the House Surgeon was pushed back to a place of disadvantage."[48] Doctors knew that, given the relatively limited number of interesting medical cases, it was essential to maximize contact with patients. The situation in the emergency room further illustrated the competition for patients. In return for hospital privileges, private doctors were required to work on the staff a few hours a week, where they came in contact with emergency and ambulance cases. The temptation was particularly strong for a doctor to admit to his own service an interesting medical case or a patient who seemed capable of paying.

Lay admitting personnel often suspected a discrepancy between a true medical emergency and what Kavanagh termed the "doctor's emergency." "Of course emergencies will arise," he noted in his discussion of the competition and distrust that existed among the staff, "but emergencies would be few if the Attendings so decreed." Kavanagh commented on the structural relations that created what he called the doctors' emergencies. "Sometimes an Attending in a very frank moment has said: 'We must get the patient in at once, or some one else will get her.' " Kavanagh felt that such "violation of rules for personal reasons by the Attendings had a demoralizing effect on the House Staff. If the Attendings consider their own personal interests first, is it any wonder that the House Staff follow their example?"[49]

When the growth in medical knowledge and expertise resulted in medical specialization, battles for control were fought on a more sophisticated level. Doctors began to argue about who had sufficient skill and medical expertise to be allowed to treat a particular patient.

At a time when there was an oversupply of physicians, the decision to specialize gave doctors a competitive advantage over their colleagues as well as a chance to learn new and interesting techniques.[50] As practitioners developed specialty interests and as associations, societies, and hospitals developed greater specialty focus, debates ensued over which physicians should be allowed to practice a specialty, how licensure accreditation for specialists should be introduced, and whether such regulation of practice should be introduced at all.[51] The American profession, unlike those of Britain and other European countries, did not make a professional distinction between physicians and surgeons. Physicians in the United States had long engaged in all forms of practice, including surgery, with little or no special training, licensure, or professional accreditation.[52] Needless to say, generalists sought to maintain their right to exclusive treatment of their patients, whereas specialists tried to lay claim to these same patients. In the medical schools and affiliated hospitals, the problems of defining who was a specialist and determining what accommodations should be made for a physician who laid claim to a specialty were especially pronounced. For example, when surgery developed into a specialty, most general practitioners were reluctant to give up the surgical part of their practice. When gynecological surgery became a subspecialty, both gynecologists and surgeons lost patients.[53]

At the Long Island College Hospital, the developing friction between the specialist surgeon and his generalist colleagues broke out in early 1900. On March 10, 1900, Henry H. Morton, a teacher at the hospital's medical school, wrote to Dr. Joseph Raymond, the secretary of the faculty of the hospital, asking for "an audience at the next meeting" of the faculty and board of regents.[54] Morton wished to be present at the meeting to protest the fact that he had been prevented from gaining clinical control over a number of patients who, in his judgment, should appropriately be placed under his care. Although he was a professor of genitourinary surgery at the medical college, he observed that he had been unable to obtain authority over patients in need of such surgery at the hospital. He complained that appropriate patients were often sent to the general surgery wards of the hospital, where the general surgeons had paid varying degrees of attention to them. "During the past five years," Morton noted, "I have done nearly every form of Genito Urinary operation, before the class [at the medical college], operating for stone in the bladder . . . performed external and internal urethroscopy for stricture, amputation of the penis for cancer; [and] castration." Furthermore, he had been "appointed to the position of Genito Urinary Surgeon to the Hospital," but because of certain general surgeons, he had not been allowed to practice his skills in the hospital. Instead of having access to genitourinary cases, he had been assigned to the Venereal Wards, where few persons in need of his surgical talents were ever placed.[55]

From Morton's perspective, the major culprit in this episode was a

Dr. DeLaTour, the chief of surgery, who had misinterpreted the conditions of Morton's appointment to the hospital. DeLaTour, Morton urged, "claimed that . . . my work was limited to the *care* of *cases* in the *Venereal Ward alone* and that he as a General Surgeon to the Hospital claimed all the Genito Urinary cases coming into the surgical wards for operation."[56]

At issue in this tiny drama was the definition and limits of the new specialty of genitourinary surgery. DeLaTour observed that specialists "had taken the Gynecology away from the [general] surgeons and if they took away the Genito Urinary Diseases too, [the general surgeon's] field would be reduced still further." For this reason he "would not be willing to give up the Genito Urinary cases."[57] Morton questioned the training of the general surgeons and insisted that the needs of medical education demanded that specialists be given control over these cases. He pointed out that "such great advances have been made in this specialty within the last few years that the subject is not adequately covered in the text books." He added, "To present it properly, demonstrations and operations upon patients are required."[58]

Indeed, there had been a tremendous advance in the skills and techniques of this important branch of surgery. Only in May 1900, a number of weeks before Morton presented his case to the hospital's board of regents, the prestigious *Philadelphia Medical Journal* wrote an editorial addressing this very issue. The journal's editors asked, "Is Genito Urinary Surgery a Specialty?" and answered with a resounding yes. "The general surgeon hates to acknowledge that any part of his field has become so highly cultivated that he must yield its care to a specialist," they remarked, but the "genito urinary tract has been the field of the most persevering study and remarkable advances in the last few years." The various instruments and techniques used in this specialty required a particular skill. The urethroscope was "as difficult to use . . . as the laryngoscope," and other instruments required great dexterity and tactile sensibility. Although it "cannot be denied that some general surgeons can use one or another of the instruments . . . both with skill and dexterity," the editors concluded that the "genito-urinary surgeon must be a specialist both in his training and his practice."[59]

When doctors could not gain control of patients by virtue of their expertise in a specialty, they sought to dominate important staff positions and often met opposition from trustees. At Methodist Hospital the board of managers responded to complaints about the inefficiency, disorganization, and dangerous practices of the surgical staff by proposing that a chief of surgical services be appointed. Rather than have surgeons fight among themselves over access to patients and facilities, the board sought to "secure greater unity in the organization and direction of the hospital" by proposing that one surgeon be on continuous service throughout the year and responsible for scheduling staff and operations. He would see that all staff members were assigned to cases for which they were appropriately trained and that younger house staff would be able to gain needed experience by assisting better-trained surgeons in their operations.[60] The superintendent argued that the present system "was working disastrously . . . in the training of Nurses and House Staff, and in the care of patients because it lacked uniformity of ideals and method which could only be brought about by having one strong man appointed as Chief or Director."[61]

The superintendent and trustees at Methodist Hospital had become especially concerned with the growing complexity and disorganization of the enlarged surgical staff because of a rash of bad publicity concerning the hospital's services. "Criticisms had been so persistent that a very large number of people in the city, and out of it, were constantly asking what was the trouble in the Hospital."[62] Many criticisms came from staff members themselves, who objected to the competition, lack of direction, and disorganization of the surgical staff. Student nurses and recent medical school graduates began to avoid service at Methodist Hospital. "One of our best nurses, who had completed more than half her course in the Training School, was requested by her uncle, a surgeon residing a thousand miles from here, to leave our Training School," observed the superintendent. "The reason for his request was that one of our Attendings had represented the organization of our surgical work as the worst possible."[63] Though some claimed that a decrease in the number of medical graduates in this period made the trustees more dependent on its house staff, others disagreed. Stated Superintendent Kavanagh, "It would be well for the Medical Board to consider if there is not a more real reason for the shortage of applicants [for house staff positions] than . . . the lack of graduates from medical colleges." He argued that young doctors were losing interest in the hospital because attending physicians were hoarding the challenging cases.[64]

Trustees also feared that the incentive for physicians to perform operations for which they were unqualified was too great to resist. Lacking an extensive private practice, most general physicians gained surgical experience with ward patients assigned to them in the hospital. Others would perform operations and other medical procedures on emergency and walk-in patients in order to keep them as private patients. Kavanagh conducted a survey of the surgical practices of the hospital's attending staff and noted that, by operating on cases for which they were unqualified, poorly prepared physicians were depriving younger physicians of "the necessary experience to make them safe and skillful in the operating room."[65]

Kavanagh's analysis showed that few of the hospital's appointed physicians performed many operations. One surgeon had referred only eight patients to the hospital in an eight-month period; another referred only five during four months. The third attending surgeon referred twenty-one patients in eight months; the fourth referred twenty-four in the same period; and the other two referred a fairly respectable number of patients upon whom the particular attending physicians could perfect their surgical skills. The superintendent noted that most of the attending surgeons had averaged between one and three operations a month – hardly enough to warrant complete confidence in their technical ability. These "analyses indicated the fact that some of the men annually appointed have not the surgical experience to be entrusted with the responsibility of a full Attending position in the Hospital. They might very well be Associates or Assistants to more experienced men, but should not be entrusted with full responsibility." The superintendent concluded that "such men need a Chief for their own good, and that of the Hospital."[66]

While the superintendent and the trustees sought to nominate a chief surgeon who would be responsible for assigning cases to trained surgeons, the surgical staff argued that such a "Surgeon in Chief is either a tyrant or a figure head." In a long letter to the trustees the surgeons charged that the trustees were attempting to appoint "a despot of [their] own creation" who would derive authority only from a lay board. "In order to successfully enact the former role [of tyrant] someone must be found who is so manifestly preeminent in comparison with his colleagues that there can be no question as to the propriety of his assumption of autocratic powers," commented Dr. J. Bion Bogart, chairman of the medical board. The surgeons maintained that they found "no such individual [among the hospital's staff] and, if we go further and scan the surgical talent of the entire borough, our search would be in vain." Continued Bogart, "To single out one [of the attending surgeons] . . . and set him in authority over the others would be so unkind to him and so unfair to each of the others that we have yet to be convinced that anyone of us would accept the position if it were offered to him." The surgeons suggested that the physicians themselves nominate a surgical "advisory member" to consult with the superintendent on problems that arose. The goal of greater "unity in the organization and direction of the surgical work," Bogart concluded, "can be secured in a very simple manner, without the slightest injustice to any individual or any disturbance of the harmonious conduct of the surgical work . . . by requesting the Attending Adult Surgical Staff to select one of their number to confer with the Superintendent upon all such matters."[67]

From the superintendent's point of view, a full-time hospital staff whose practices and interests would revolve solely around the hospital would guarantee a commitment to the efficient functioning of the hospital. Furthermore, by guaranteeing those few physicians a substantial portion of walk-in or emergency cases, the hospital could rest assured that its surgeons were at least gaining the skill necessary to be effective surgeons. Because there were too few interesting or significant surgical patients – walk-in or private – to provide the enlarged staff with an adequate number of cases for training, Kavanagh proposed to limit the attending physicians to practice on their own private patients and to assisting the chief on walk-ins.

The attending surgeons objected to the chief of service's being given first choice of cases that came through the emergency admissions and dispensary. They feared that this arrangement would limit their ability to secure enough private patients to keep them working regularly at any but the most mundane tasks. As members of the enlarged hospital staff, these physicians recognized that there were already too few patients to support more than a small number of full-time staff members, but they wanted at least *equal* access to walk-in patients.[68]

Although the initial confrontations between doctors and administrators led to a standoff, ultimately a compromise plan of reorganization was worked out. To prevent doctors from politicking individually over admitting patients, two surgical services were organized – each headed by a surgeon. This arrangement centralized authority over the distribution of patients without limiting power in this area to one individual. Because the selection of the two head surgeons was made by the attending surgeons themselves, with the approval of the executive board, there was little chance that they would exert power independently of the medical personnel.[69]

This compromise solution indicated the growing power and authority of the medical personnel in the hospital. By early 1915 physicians at Methodist Hospital were making policy for themselves and contradicting the policy and intentions of the lay board. "Communications at different times have been received from the Medical Board which indicate that the [Medical] Board has taken certain matters into their hands which belong to the [lay] Board of Managers," reported the executive committee in February 1915. The lay board objected to a new rule adopted by the doctors "by which new members of the Medical Board shall be elected," and complained that the doctors "have also proceeded to accept the resignation of an Attending Obstetrician, who did not forward his resignation to the Board of Managers, the body which elected him." The executive committee noted that the Medical Board then nominated this obstetrician's successor, another irregular proceeding, and added that the lay board "itself should respond to [the problem] for if this sort of thing is not corrected promptly, it will grow to greater embarrassment."[70] While trustees felt that doctors were taking too much into their own hands, they could do little to stop this trend.

Conscious of their own growing professional unity and reinforced by the reform efforts of the Progressive era, doctors came to assume more and more power in the field of health care and began to win substantial victories within the hospital itself. At Methodist Hospital they succeeded in gaining the right to nominate their own representatives to the board of trustees, and they thwarted the trustees' plan to *appoint* a chief on continuous service. Having persuaded the trustees to compromise on the issue of one continuous service, they succeeded in placing their own representatives at the head of a new, dual surgical service.

By March 1915, the physicians at Methodist Hospital had assumed the authority to nominate and reject physicians for attending staff positions. The medical board passed a resolution stating that "all candidates for vacancies on the Attending Staff shall be nominated at a regular meeting of the Medical Board [and acted upon by ballots] at the next meeting." The successful candidates were then "referred to the joint committee . . . and finally to the Board of Managers for appointment."[71] As the secretary of the executive committee pointed out in a letter to the doctors, this method for choosing the new attending physicians did "not conform to the By-Laws of the [Lay] Board of Managers," which stated that the authority to nominate and accept new attending staff resided with the board of managers, not with the physicians. In fact, the entire procedure for nominating new physicians had always resided with the trustees, who were the elite members of Brooklyn society. "Doubtless by inadvertence," the managers diplomatically noted, the physicians had "over-looked" this rule, and the "secretary of the Board was requested to call the attention of the Medical Board" to the oversight.[72] Only four months earlier, the superintendent had warned the physicians that they "were on the Staff by appointment of the Board of Managers but [that] it did not follow that they had a perpetual right to the various positions."[73] By

1914 such threats had no effect because doctors had become absolutely crucial to the effective functioning of the institution.

As we have seen, the Progressive era hospital underwent tremendous organizational and ideological shifts. An institution run and organized along the lines of a paternalist charity was transformed into a highly complex bureaucracy in which medical services were bought and sold. Trustees, seeking to modernize and stabilize financially troubled institutions, found themselves forced to hand real power over to private practitioners who had little or no interest in the paternalistic goals of the older charity hospital. By 1915 doctors at many institutions had essentially wrested control from the trustees and had gained the power to make the decisions that were in their own best interests, regardless of the traditional charity goals of the hospital.

5   Taking control: political reform and hospital governance

Although internal economic and organizational struggles altered the structure of many turn-of-the-century hospitals, some changes were the result of new policies in city government. Changes made during this era in the system of municipal reimbursement to the hospital have remained important until today and have had significant long-term effects. Local control and some forms of decision making passed from hospital trustees and their ward boss representatives to city administrators, who defined more narrowly the hospital work they would reimburse. Ultimately, changes in the municipal reimbursement system resulted in a loss of autonomy for many hospitals and a loss of funds so severe that some were forced out of existence.

The Tammany machine and flat-grant payments for charity

In the years after the Civil War, control over New York's political machinery moved to the infamous Tammany Hall led by Mayor William Marcy Tweed, Richard Croker, and Charles F. Murphy. With only brief interruptions totaling ten years, Tammany politicians controlled the mayor's office, the administrative machinery, and the patronage jobs of New York's government for nearly three-quarters of a century. Unlike the later Progressives, who appealed for financial support to the upper- and middle-class populations of the city's neighborhoods, the Tammany machine based its power on its ability to gain political support from the working populations of highly diverse communities. Tammany's power was its local ward structure and, most particularly, the ability of its ward boss to gather votes and support in his district. George Washington Plunkitt, the colorful Tammany ward boss from New York's West Side, showed how a Tammany Hall politician maintained power when he said that a politician, to hold his district, must "study human nature and act accordin'." He announced in the early 1900s: "I know every man, woman and child in the Fifteenth District, except them that's been born this Summer . . . I know what they like and what they don't like,, what they are strong at and what they are weak in, and I reach them by approachin' at the right side."[1]

Vol. IX, No. 6
June, 1920

HOSPITAL
MANAGEMENT

417 S. Dearborn
Street,
Chicago

Published in the Interest of Executives in Every Department of Hospital Work

Something in Both Hands

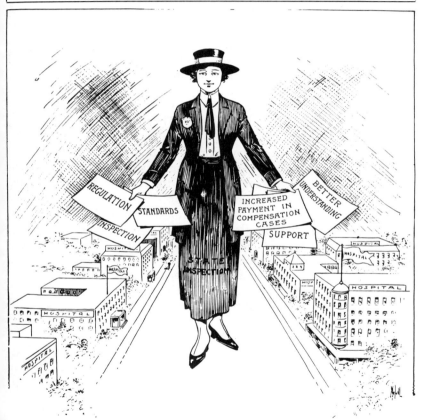

The growing role of the state in regulating the activities of the hospital met with some resistance. Here *Hospital Management* points out that "State Inspection" is bringing "Something in Both Hands." Among the factors balancing regulations, standards, and inspection was, not insignificantly, increased payment in compensation cases.

The power of the local ward boss rested largely in his ability to respond to the practical problems of his district quickly and personally. By doing so he gained the trust and personal allegiance necessary to maintain political control over the district and to ensure the political power of the Tammany organization overall. "What tells in holdin' your grip on your district is to go right down among the poor families and help them in the different ways they need help," Plunkitt stated.

> If there's a fire in Ninth, Tenth, or Eleventh Avenue, for example, any hour of the day or night, I'm usually there with some of my election district captains as soon as the fire engines . . . If a family is burned out I don't ask whether they are Republicans or Democrats and I don't refer them to the Charity Organization Society, which would investigate their case in a month or two and decide they were worthy of help about the time they are dead from starvation.

He would instead "just get quarters for them, buy clothes . . . and fix them up till they get things runnin' again."[2]

This kind of locally based political organization made sense during a time when the city's communities could maintain order and provide services with a certain amount of ease.[3] Throughout the nineteenth century small institutions that did not have enough patrons to provide them with substantial monetary support could depend upon the merchants, clergy, and other locally prominent persons who were members of the board of trustees to turn to the local ward boss; he, in exchange for political support, would use his influence to obtain grants-in-aid from the city treasury. These grants were provided annually to institutions on the condition that they be used solely to support charitable activities. With no requirements for reporting or justifying the way the funds were spent, the flat-grant system made possible the continued existence of the small charity facilities and also provided the necessary charity services not offered by the city. By unwritten agreement, the city provided funds on the condition that the hospitals and dispensaries care for the working poor in whatever ways were necessary.

Until the Depression of the 1890s this system worked fairly well, at least well enough not to be or be seen as a severe problem. Small charity facilities did what they wished, and ultimately it worked out that some provided ambulance and emergency services, some maternity services, some food and shelter for the homeless. In the 1840s Kings County Hospital was organized as an adjunct to the almshouse, thereby becoming the only public hospital in Brooklyn. Kings County was a formidable distance from the city's population center and was therefore of limited use to the city's working class and nonindigent patients.

Because the County hospital served a clientele largely indistinguishable from the almshouse inmates, it had little appeal to nonindigent working-class patients who shunned the stigma of the almshouse. In addition, by mid-century, city authorities realized that more public services were needed and that Kings County was too far away for many people needing immediate care. City officials began to develop formal and informal mechanisms to provide hospital care for public patients by funding the private charity hospitals already located in central parts of the city. Charity institutions like the Brooklyn City Hospital, often referred to simply as "City Hospital," were generally thought of as public facilities, when in fact they were actually private institutions independent of municipal authority or control.[4]

Whenever the demand for services for the indigent, for the homeless, or for emergency patients increased, the city simply gave more funds to the private charitable institutions already in existence. "When the city authorities first took up the question of caring for homeless and destitute persons . . . some of the private charitable institutions were already in existence and came forward with offers to share the burden," observed one reformer in 1901. Though "at the time it was considered a good business arrangement for the city to use private societies," this writer felt that "by giving money to private persons . . . they invited the creation of new societies and a steadily increasing demand for new funds."[5]

By the late nineteenth century, the number of independent charities receiving public funds had grown so much that what had been a contractual convenience became a major city enterprise. Generally the city had not kept track of services in distant sections. By 1897, the year before the incorporation of Greater New York, the City of Brooklyn alone provided partial support for sixty-two charitable institutions and societies. Of these, twenty-four were general and specialty hospitals that received subsidies ranging from $2,000 to $5,000; twenty-one others were dispensaries that received a standard payment of $1,500 directly from the city.[6] There were few criteria regulating the distribution of these funds. Small temporary dispensaries like the Twenty-sixth Ward Homeopathic Dispensary received the same $1,500 grant as did the larger, well-established facilities like the Long Island College Dispensary. One small hospital was awarded a $4,000 stipend although the aldermen were not sure of its real name.[7] A wide range of medical services, missionary societies, and soup kitchens received the same appropriations as did large hospitals and established dispensaries. For example, Brooklyn Diet Dispensary, the Brooklyn Eclectic Dispensary, the Gates Avenue Homeopathic Dispensary, and St. Phoebe's Mission were reimbursed at the same rate as the Long Island College Hospital, Brooklyn City Hospital, and Methodist Episcopal Hospital. Though larger institutions did not depend on the city stipend, the smaller institutions did. John T. Wells, secretary of the small Bedford Dispensary and Hospital, noted in its 1898 *Annual Report* the important role of public appropriations in the facility when he observed that it had grown "from a small institution supported wholly by private charity to its present position as a public benefaction largely supported by public taxation."[8]

The apparently arbitrary nature by which funds were disbursed during the mid-nineteenth century reflected real problems in the organization of communication in the growing city. Nineteenth-century Brooklyn, as noted in Chapter 1, was large and geographically diverse. Communication was hampered by the lack of a telephone system, a rapid transit system, and even a decent roadbed. As a result, city officials were largely dependent on information provided to them by special ward or local interests. Yearly flat grants were provided to diverse services for the very good reason that it was difficult or impossible to differentiate between kinds of services and impossible to maintain close supervision over these services. Because there were few methods by which government could keep track of the needs of its rapidly growing population, public funding of private charity seemed to ensure the distribution of services in newly developed areas distant from city hall. City government, on the one hand, benefited from the fact that private agencies were willing to take on the responsibility of providing emergency services that the city was unable to offer in any rational way; emergency room care, ambulance service, and housing for the poor or displaced were forms of assistance essential to the city's smooth functioning. Local charity, on the other hand, had the benefit of reimbursement by the city for services that it would otherwise have to provide itself.

The inadequacies of this loosely organized system became apparent by the end of the century. Throughout the 1890s there were serious debates over how to improve an ambulance service that was, at the height of the Depression, proving to be extremely inadequate. In 1895 the health commissioner of Brooklyn wrote to the superintendents of the city's hospitals asking them to improve their emergency services. "Although the accusation of inhumanity, occasionally made against the hospital authorities and ambulance surgeons of the city, is generally undeserved," he maintained, "it must, nevertheless, be admitted that, unfortunately, such is not always the case." He was upset that there were certain "well authenticated instances of patients . . . having been refused transportation by ambulance surgeons," as well as cases in which patients had been "denied admission to hospitals which are under contract with the city to care for the sick and poor." The commissioner was concerned that the hospitals were not fulfilling their obligations to the city, and he sought to legislate compliance from the charity organizations. "The hospital that is under contract with the city to treat the sick poor," he stated, "must maintain an emergency ward . . . for the temporary reception of ambulance cases." Furthermore, "this ward is to be used for no other purposes." He also demanded that "cases of grave injury or sickness must be admitted even when brought from another district."[9]

The Depression had greatly altered the situation of the city and upset the previous balance between community need and charity services. Many more people than before were homeless, poor, and in need of services. Charity hospitals were limited in their ability to care for the homeless and indigent, the alcoholics, and the growing population of vagrants who were often the people brought in by ambulance. Because these hospitals had always seen their goal as caring for the "worthy" poor, they could send the so-called unworthy poor elsewhere without altering their perception of their goal. In their opinion the growing number of homeless people were the responsibility of the police department, the prison, or the public hospital. Although this had always been the belief of the charity hospitals, in the past they had found it easier to absorb the smaller number of vagrants and alcoholics who were picked up by their ambulance services. With the increased poverty and illness brought on by the Depression, the hospitals began to restrict their services by seeking ways to identify more accurately the needy working-class or "worthy" poor. This policy left many city administrators feeling that, even though the city paid out funds to small charity hospitals to care for the homeless and those in need of emergency services, they were not being cared for to a sufficient extent.

It became clear that no comprehensive reform would come from the charity institutions themselves. They were long used to arranging services as they saw fit, with no specific expectations from the city. Furthermore, they were doing their best to survive during hard times. If they could receive money from benefactors for offering particular services, they would offer these services even if an outside city administrator might see far more need for emergency services in the community. If there were a chance of receiving some income from working-class patients through direct payments they would be reluctant to use their services primarily for emergency, and ambulance cases who might not ever contribute to the institution. Their concern was not the overall efficient functioning of the system but the survival of their own facilities. By the end of the century, there were serious conflicts between the city, which sought comprehensive reform, and a charity system that appeared to be breaking down.

Progressive reforms and the charity system

The shape taken by changes in the provision of charity services was largely determined by the goals of the Progressive era reformers who came to power at the end of the nineteenth century. By the closing years of the century, the Progressives were in a battle with the ward bosses of the Democratic Party machine for control of the city.[10] In nearly every area of urban life, Progressive reformers sought to undermine the authority, legitimacy, and political power of locally elected ward bosses who traditionally controlled city contracts, public jobs, and services in immigrant communities. In New York and other American cities, Progressives sought to gain control of local city appointments by appealing to the governor or other state representatives farther removed from local political struggles. Reformers also sought to replace the older aldermanic system of ward-based city elections with a city manager system and a council elected on a city-wide basis.[11] Uniformly, the tools of the Progressive reformer were regulation and administration through the offices of centralized government. Unlike reformers of earlier years, who sought to return to a simpler time, Progressives looked forward to a day when expertise would be harnessed to control a complex new industrial world.

By the end of the century a battle between reformers and supporters of the local political machine was inevitable, and much was at stake. After all, the 1898 incorporation of the cities of New York and Brooklyn had created the nation's largest and wealthiest city. Control over city government meant control over patronage, jobs, city planning, contracts, and the commercial development of the city. From the perspective of the reformers, Tammany Hall was composed of corrupt, primarily immigrant politicians whose inefficiency interfered with the city's economic and commercial growth. But Tammany politicians saw reformers as "morning glories" who knew little about politics and less about people. "The fact is that a reformer can't last in politics," reported Tammany's Plunkitt. A reformer "might make a splurge for a while, as long as his money lasted," but he could be counted on to make "a mess of it every time."[12]

The civil service law, a central and favorite of Progressives, was an attack on the patronage system crucial to the maintenance of the Tammany machine. To Plunkitt, civil service reform was "the biggest fraud of the age" and "the curse of the nation." It was a curse that undermined the country, patriotism, and of course the Tammany machine. "Just look at things in the city today," he exclaimed. "There are ten thousand good offices, but we can't get at more than a few hundred of them." Plunkitt asked, "How are we goin' to provide for the thousands of men who worked for the Tammany ticket?" and answered his own question: "It can't be done." The net effect of the reformers' civil service law was a little short of catastrophic from Plunkitt's view: He related that he knew "more than one young man . . . who worked for the [Tammany] ticket and was just overflowing with patriotism, but when he was knocked out by the civil service humbug he got to hate his country and became an Anarchist."[13]

The displacement of Tammany by the Progressives essentially meant that power was passing from a locally controlled political system long associated with the working class to a government of Progressives whose alliance was with professionals and business people interested in gaining control of a city government that had been lost to immigrants in the preceding decades. By presenting programs that promised to put rationality and order into the life of a seemingly chaotic city, Progressives were able to win the support of those business people and professionals who had a stake in a smooth-running system of government and city services. Reformers would generally win election to public office by challenging the ability of locally elected ward bosses to deliver services and jobs to their constituencies. By setting up state- and city-wide standards for public service positions in the form of a civil service system, they undermined the local ward boss's ability to give jobs to his political allies. Progressive reformers also proposed an increase in the power of disinterested expert commissions and panels appointed by central office managers. This change effectively diluted the local boss's ability to influence the city's political life. Employing the business person's vision of the productive capacity of large industrial plants organized around bureaucratic administrations, reformers were quick to view larger hospitals as more productive and efficient than smaller ones.[14] This vision gave little heed to the ability of communities to make crucial decisions on their own and ultimately caused the demise of some local community institutions.

One of the men central to the Progressive reform of the charity system was Bird S. Coler. "By some good fortune there was nominated in 1897 for the office of Comptroller of the enlarged city of New York . . . a young man unknown in politics named Bird S. Coler," declared an 1899 editorial in the *Independent*, a New York reform weekly.[15] Born in Champaign, Illinois, on October 9, 1867, Coler was raised in Brooklyn. His father, who owned a brokerage firm, sent him to Brooklyn's public schools and then to Philips Academy. After graduation he entered his father's brokerage house and made money on the rising Northern Pacific Railroad.[16] He soon became involved in Brooklyn politics and lost his first bid for public office in 1894. In 1897 Coler succeeded in gaining a place as comptroller on the mayoral ticket of Robert Van Wyck, the Tammany Hall politician. In the year before incorporation, Tammany Boss Richard Croker sought to solidify his authority over the new Borough of Brooklyn by creating a variety of political linkages between Brooklyn and New York.[17] Croker picked Coler to run for comptroller because Coler was a young man unknown in the world of New York politics. "Those who inquired as to his history were told that he was a resident of Brooklyn and had been associated with his father in a banking house, where he had learned something about municipal bonds," reported the *Independent*. "With this they were forced to be content." Coler's youth, inexperience, and Brooklyn residency were major factors in his 1897 nomination.[18] Although dependence on Tammany Hall would be intermittent, Coler in fact owed his political beginning to the Tammany machine.

Coler's ambitions soon went beyond the office of comptroller. Sensing the importance of the Progressive movement, Coler sought to establish a base of power among those reformers who could support his campaigns, independent of Tammany. Upon entering office he made quick alliances with civic reformers, first in opposition to the Tammany-proposed Ramapo Water contract. Coler discovered that the Ramapo Water Company sought to swindle the city out of nearly $5 million; the company, in fact, had a mere $5,000 in assets and little equipment with which to guarantee the delivery of two hundred million gallons of water a day. By exposing collusion between Ramapo Water and Tammany members on the Board of Public Improvements, Coler gained the enmity of Tammany and the affection of the clean-government reformers. "He has neglected no opportunity . . . to protect the city treasury," noted the *Independent*. "It was due to his fearless determined opposition that the purpose of the Tammany office-holders to commit the city to the Ramapo Water Contract was thwarted – a contract involving the payment in forty years of more than $200,000,000 to a company which was controlled by politicians and had not a reservoir, a pump, or a pipe."[19]

Coler's second major act as comptroller was to reorder the mechanisms by which the city disbursed public funds to charity facilities. In
1899 a bill was introduced and passed by the state legislature, amend-
ing New York City's charter so that the city's government became
solely responsible for the distribution of municipal funds to all charitable institutions. Known as the Stranahan bill in honor of the state
senator from Brooklyn who introduced it, this piece of legislation was,
declared Coler, "destined to revolutionize the relations existing between the city treasury and private eleemosynary institutions."[20] In an
article in *Popular Science*, Coler noted: "The last legislature passed a bill
placing in the hands of the local Board of Estimate absolute power over
all appropriations for charitable purposes, and for the first time in
many years reform is possible."[21]

At the heart of Coler's proposed reforms was his desire to regularize
the methods by which charity institutions were held accountable to
the public. He viewed the former system of flat grants to institutions
sponsored by local ward representatives as inefficient, in that no one
really kept track of the money and its uses. "The giving of public
money in lump sums . . . of which there is no public or official inspection, should be discontinued at once," he stated. "I shall urge that all
appropriations to institutions of every kind not controlled by the city
be limited to per capita payments for the support of public charities,
and that a system of thorough inspection be at once established to
ascertain if present and future inmates are really persons entitled to
maintenance at public expense." Coler specifically warned charity institutions that they should not expect public support unless they could
account to the city: The "comptroller should have full power to with-
hold payments to any institution after an appropriation has been made
if in his judgment, after examination, the money has not been earned."[22]
To ensure observation of the new rules, inspectors from the Department of Public Charities verified the institutions' requests and visited
these facilities to help organize their inspection and accounting procedures. In addition, a separate bureau was organized in the comptroller's
office for the collection of data and "for subsequent revision or modifi-
cation of the rules."[23]

The per diem, per capita system of reimbursement was far more
powerful than the flat-grant system in guiding reluctant hospitals to
adopt the goals of the city. By inspecting the social conditions, class,
and medical criteria of each patient, and reimbursing hospitals only for
clients deemed "appropriate," the city was able to force community
institutions to meet certain minimal standards in their admissions policies. Whereas charity hospitals had once received funds irrespective of

how they used them, after Coler they were paid only for doing the specific work the city wanted done. Generally, this meant providing ambulance and emergency services to people the small hospitals might have tended to shun as "unworthy."

Coler implied that there had previously been no criteria for dispensing money. Though in some sense he was correct, his moves toward regulation were problematical: Who established the standards for institutions? Was the purpose of regulation only to fund institutions, or was it also to guarantee quality services to patients? It is important to remember that hospitals had grown up in response to local and highly distinct perceptions of community needs. As such, small institutions had little in common with each other in accounting techniques, admission policies, or even the social characteristics of their patients. To standardize reimbursement policies for such a diversity of institutions was extremely arbitrary in and of itself. Generally the standards that were adopted were not those of the smallest, least powerful institutions.

Coler's reforms reflected a deep belief in the viability of municipal government and the need to reform its means of operation. In his book *Municipal Government*, he observed that the last quarter of the nineteenth century had witnessed the rapid growth of the American city and a corresponding growth in the complexity of the issues faced by government officials: No "graver problems of government exist . . . than those developed during the last quarter of the nineteenth century in the management of [city] affairs." Tremendous change had occurred in the "principles of finance, education, charity, public health, and politics," and the responsibilities of public officials and government agencies had also changed. "The time when city government was supposed to consist of a mayor and alderman elected to perform certain arbitrary and ornamental duties" was past. The "proper government of cities has at last come to be recognized as a work of broader scope than maintaining streets and highways, preserving order, and collecting taxes to pay the bills." Now government was responsible for creating an organized whole out of the individual interests of the city's residents. The administrator, the expert, and the bureaucrat adopted the ideals of business and efficiency in order to manage a complex and heterogeneous metropolis. "Everywhere," Coler noted, "there is a promising tendency toward thorough business methods in the conduct of the affairs of the cities."[24]

Coler saw his goals and methods as far different from those of the earlier reformers. He observed that many reformers, "when they enter politics, present platforms built of . . . platitudes which . . . mean something like this: 'We would suppress gambling and the social evil, eradicate vice of all kinds, enforce all Sunday laws, make the city good and virtuous by force, reduce expenditures and taxation and conduct the public business honestly and cheaply.' " Coler found these goals vague and pious and "impossible to a very large extent until human nature itself is changed." In contrast, he considered that modern reform required a "broad and liberal policy for building up, not a mere negative force to stop progress in order to show a smaller expense account."[25]

Coler's intention was to replace the informal and personalized mechanisms by which city funds were distributed prior to his assumption of office with formal procedures regulated by city government. When he entered the comptroller's office in 1898, he "found that the city officers were practically powerless" and that there "had been no attempt at regulation or reform [of the system of disbursement] for thirty years." An investigation of the charity system in New York City convinced him "that the city should have absolute control over all appropriations to private societies and institutions." He maintained that the old charity system had allowed the institutions and their ward bosses to judge their own needs, and that this system promoted waste, inefficiency, and, at times, corruption. He pointed out that the personalized relationships between city officials and local charity administrators had led to "gross inequalities" in the funds disbursed to different institutions providing services.[26]

Coler was not merely tightening up the system as he claimed. In many ways he began to view regulation as a way to ensure that small, independent facilities provided only those services not provided elsewhere. In a certain sense he was changing the rules of the game. For many years charity hospitals had been reimbursed for offering whatever services were needed by the public and not available at a local public hospital. When Coler took office a number of large public hospitals were in place, and others were being planned, so that it was cheaper for the city to finance patients in public hospitals than in small independent facilities. The city was reluctant to fund small facilities by means of flat grants for fear that the city would be supporting patients who could pay while the beds in the public hospital remained empty.

Coler was convinced that patients needing long-term or planned acute care could use the public hospitals. But he recognized that the city could not afford to support emergency and ambulance services throughout the city and that the small charity institutions could still be used to provide such services. After all, these small institutions were already in place in areas too far from the public hospitals in the case of an emergency.[27]

Unfortunately, as we have seen, small, private facilities did not see their role in this way. They were moving toward the provision of planned care for paying patients in order to make up the deficit in hospital income caused by the decrease in funds from the city. They were thinking about expanding their private services, not their services for the indigent, in part because the city reimbursement for services to the poor was insufficient to cover their expenses.

The response to Coler's hospital reimbursement system

Coler's reform of the mechanism for hospital reimbursement had immediate and long-term effects. According to his new system, hospitals were to be reimbursed at a standard rate of sixty cents per day for medical cases and eighty cents per day for surgical cases accepted by city inspectors. A lump sum of eighteen dollars was paid for maternity cases. The mechanism was simple but required the institutions to develop new administrative and organizational structures: The hospital's administrator or physician submitted the names of patients thought to be appropriate "city cases" to the Department of Public Charities, or, in Brooklyn, to the Bureau of Charities. The department's eight investigators then examined social, economic, and residency characteristics of the patients and determined their appropriateness as public charges.[28]

This system of reimbursement severely limited the funds available to small institutions. Whereas the old flat-grant system guaranteed a set amount of money every year, the new system made institutions largely dependent upon the determinations of individual inspectors who visited their facilities. Because smaller institutions had relatively few beds, they received less money under the per capita method of payment than under the old system. Even if all their patients were accepted as city charges, maximum payment was limited because of the small number of patients the hospital could house. "Owing to change in the Department of Charities, we realized early in this year that we were not to receive our usual city appropriations," lamented an administrator at Brooklyn's Nursery and Infants' Hospital who had failed to screen his patients closely enough. "This had not been foreseen, so no effort to make good the deficit had been made. Our Treasury being depleted, we were obliged to *borrow* money to meet our expenses."[29] At Brooklyn Hospital, as well, the trustees lamented the change in city reimbursement. "The most important incident of the year, affecting the financial part of our work," declared John Leech, president of the hospital, "was the promulgation by the Comptroller of the City of New York of new, elaborate, and somewhat complex rules regarding the distribution of the appropriations made to charitable institutions by the city." Leech feared that the income from the city would diminish at the very time when the costs of the facility were rising. "The cost of caring for our charity patients during 1899 was more than three times the amount received from the city for that period," he pointed out. If, in the future, "the income from the city is to be reduced, the Trustees must seek for still larger benefactions from the already overtaxed charitable citizens of Brooklyn."[30]

At Brooklyn Eye and Ear, "the new method put in vogue . . . for the distribution of city funds . . . diminished the revenues of the hospital $1,577." While acknowledging that Coler might have reason to complain about the arbitrary nature of hospital admitting procedures, the chairman of the board of trustees still protested that the reality injured clients and institutions alike. "In the abstract, the principle of distribution according to the number of days a poor patient is boarding in a hospital may be just and wise, but the concrete application of it has caused not a little embarrassment to some of the beneficiaries of the city."[31] Similarly, at Methodist Episcopal Hospital, the change in payment also brought immediate concern. "Our revenue for the year has not been adequate," observed the superintendent. "There are various explanations [one of which is that payments] by the City of New York for the work which we have done for the sick poor have not been as liberal as heretofore."[32]

Although all institutions complained, the smaller institutions suffered most. When the small Williamsburg Hospital made a last-ditch appeal for charitable bequests in January 1903, its president, D. M. Munger, explained that the "reasons for the [poor] financial conditions of the institution [were the] increased cost of maintenance and [the cut in] city appropriations."[33] Three days later, the Williamsburg Hospital "closed its doors . . . for lack of funds."[34] D. C. Potter, the chief examiner of accounts of the city's finance department, reported to the Board of Estimate that many charitable institutions were "bordering on financial panic." He recommended that the "per capita appropriation by the city for patients in such places be increased. Managers of hospitals . . . [have] stated . . . that they were confronting the necessity of closing their doors and turning their patients and wards back to the mercies of the city."[35]

Trustees of many smaller institutions were most upset over the loss of funds, but some also objected to implicit changes in the relationship between the city and the independent hospitals. Methodist Hospital's president was particularly perplexed about these changes. "A certain amount of work is done in every hospital which is properly chargeable to the city," he observed. The consolidation of Brooklyn and Manhattan had disrupted the older pattern of flat-grant payment, in which his hospital had "more than earned its appropriation." Under the new plan, a city inspector "from the commissioner visits the Hospital and interviews [our] patient." Then the investigator decided upon payment. Even "if the cases are approved by the inspector they may be rejected by the commissioner. And the result is that though a larger quantity of work is done for the city's poor than under the old plan . . . the Hospital receives less money than before." He objected to the method by which the city decided on the amount of money to be reimbursed: "In the first place our Hospital is not similar to the city hospitals." It was unfair for the city to compare the private charity facilities to the city facilities. "An allowance of eighty or sixty cents may be adequate for a day's support of . . . patients in a city hospital," he observed, "but we spend thrice the lesser amount [for the care of our patients]."[36]

Implicit in the trustees' objections to the new city regulations were the fears that a new, unnecessary bureaucracy might develop and that city bureaucrats might, for the first time, challenge the authority of the trustees by involving themselves in the inner workings and administration of the charity hospitals. With the city's new emphasis on accountability and per diem, per capita payments, city inspectors were already involved in the day-to-day routine of the hospital – interviewing patients, reviewing the hospital's accounting system, and, most important, evaluating the hospital's administrative and professional staff. Methodist and other independent hospitals wished to return to the former method of flat-grant payment in order to maintain distance between themselves and the city. "I am convinced," noted Methodist's president, "that the thing to do is for the city to make contracts with certain hospitals . . . and pay them according to contract."[37]

The Charity Organization Society reacted to the city's actions, but for substantially different reasons. Though impressed by the city's efforts to introduce "system and uniformity" into hospital record keeping, the society feared that an open-ended system of per capita payments might allow too much rather than too little city money for the larger independent hospitals. "Several institutions which received only very small appropriations and were chiefly supported by private donations [will] now receive public pay for a large part of the work which they do," reported an editorial in the society's *Annual Report* of June 1900. The society thought that the unlimited per capita, per diem payments could eventually lead to a city subsidy system that would supplant and replace private charitable giving: "The question arises whether the amount dispersed prior to the adoption of the present rules should not [be] regarded as a maximum. Otherwise it will be only a very few years until public subsidies have entirely supplanted private charity in the field of medical relief."[38] Organized charity aimed to place limits on public benevolence for fear that a subsidy system might undermine the influence of private organized charity over large institutions.

The transition to the new system created a great deal of tension within the departments of the city government itself. "It was my misfortune to be placed in charge of this [new] system, in the Boroughs of Brooklyn and Queens on January 1, 1900," remarked Jesse T. Duryea, superintendent of the Kings County Hospital and Brooklyn's director of charity operations.[39] Commissioner Simis, of Brooklyn's Bureau of Charities, was verbally attacked by members of the city's new accounting department, who found "the absolute lack of system [in Simis's office was] so bad that it took two men two weeks to locate . . . orders and requisitions."[40]

Not everyone was upset by the change in reimbursement procedure, however. Those responsible for protecting the public's purse saw the new administrative organization of the Department of Public Charity and the comptroller's office as a necessary and important reform. The "ease of obtaining city funds without an accounting led some hospitals into the habit of caring for public patients that the city was not called upon to care for," observed Duryea in his critique of the city reforms. It "also encouraged a lack of effort on the part of some hospitals to force a payment from those patients who were able to pay a minimum hospital rate."[41]

Even some hospitals recognized the positive long-term effects of the changed administrative arrangements. Administrators of the Brooklyn Eye and Ear Hospital originally questioned the wisdom of the changed arrangements, but soon began to thank city officials for their help in regularizing accounting procedures and differentiating among patients who could and could not pay for hospital care. In 1901 the hospital's clinics reported "a falling off in attendance" of about 10 percent when compared with previous years. The hospital attributed this change to the effect of the dispensary law and the changed city requirements for reimbursements. "Seven hundred and thirty two have been refused treatment by the Registrar as unworthy objects of charity," noted the superintendent. Furthermore, the new regulations pertaining to charity patients "have become so widely disseminated that, doubtless, very many more have been deterred from applying for treatment." The Eye and Ear Hospital, like other facilities that still defined themselves strictly as charities, came to see the new city regulations as making the institution more efficient in serving the ends for which it had been built – the treatment of truly indigent clients: "The thanks of the Board are due and are cordially given to Mr. Nichols, Superintendent of the Bureau of Charities, for his very cordial cooperation and assistance in investigating doubtful cases . . . thus relieving the hospital of considerable expense and embarrassment."[42] The next year the Brooklyn Eye and Ear superintendent repeated his thanks for the help given by the Bureau of Charities: "Due diligence has been given to the sifting, so far as practicable, the unworthy from the worthy [recipients of charity care]. Grateful recognition is again made of the cooperation of the Bureau of Charities in the attainment of the above end. As the result of this discrimination 666 applicants for special treatment were rejected as not proper objects of charity." Similar thanks were annually offered to the city for aid in regularizing the workings of the hospital in the application of "scientific charity."[43]

Private practitioners welcomed Coler's reforms because they eased the competition for new patients. In the aftermath of the severe depression of the 1890s, many patients who could no longer afford private practitioners had begun to use the less expensive charity facilities. During this time, both the number of graduates from New York medical schools and the number of hospitals and dispensaries had grown, so that competition for paying patients was inevitable. Doctors feared that many persons and families of marginal means would abandon the relatively expensive care of community practitioners and turn to charity institutions, but Coler's reforms ensured that these people would be declared ineligible for the charity services on the grounds that they were not needy enough. As we have already noted, many of these people of marginal means were asked to pay for the services they had once received for little or no cost in the charity hospitals. As a result, charity institutions ceased to be a free alternative to expensive doctors' care, and private physicians could count on more patients. "Comptroller Coler . . . is to be heartily thanked for his efforts to minimize the abuse by which private charities are supported out of the public treasury," noted the lead editorial in the *Brooklyn Medical Journal* for November 1899. "Coming into direct antagonism with some of the most powerful organizations of our large cities he needs not only plenty of pluck and courage . . . but the hearty cooperation of all who agree with him and who have in their efforts hitherto been unsuccessful."[44] Arthur Jacobsen, another Brooklyn physician, wrote the lead article in the April 1900 issue of the *Brooklyn Medical Journal*; there he reminded doctors that they owed this reform to a businessman, not a physician: "Medical men should not forget . . . that this one great practical reform has not come through them. It has remained for practical business men of the types of Controller Coler . . . to institute it."[45]

Hospital physicians and administrators who discussed "abuse" in the health system were generally referring to the fact that individual working- and middle-class persons used charity services intended only for "the poor" and indigent – "abuse" was defined as an individual act by some unworthy recipient of public largesse. As Coler and other city officials saw it, the administrators of an institution abused charity when they allowed the use of charity services by unworthy recipients. "The chief abuses of the present system," wrote Coler, "are the extravagant expenditures for salaries [and] the misdirected efforts of the inexperienced persons who control so many of the smaller societies that receive city money."[46] In addition, Coler found that city money was not being spent to pay for services to the needy, but was being used "to pay off mortgage indebtedness . . . additions to buildings . . . increase of investments and endowment. In one case the manager of an institution frankly explained a remarkable falling off in disbursements . . . by stating that it was proposed, by exercising a great economy . . . to let the city's appropriations . . . accumulate into a respectable building fund."[47]

To Coler, corruption and inexperience were far greater abuses than were attempts by poor or working-class people to take advantage of a loose, inefficient system. As a representative of the larger Progressive movement, Coler saw accounting, accountability, and professional administration as the mechanisms by which social problems could be rationalized and reformed.[48] Because the Progressives had little confidence in decisions made by their local constituents, they felt that only an alteration of the *system* could rectify abuses.[49]

The changes in the reimbursement mechanism reflected a major change in the responsibilities of city and private charity for care of the city's poor and ill. Coler and other city officials saw the independent hospitals as an appendage to the city almshouses and public charities system. Historically, as Coler often pointed out, the independent facilities had received public funds because of the city's own inability to provide adequate services. Sometimes hospitals were funded to absorb the overflow from the public hospitals. Lewis Pilcher noted in an early critique of the city–private relationship that this relationship went "back to October 24, 1840 [when] the Superintendents of the Poor informed the Board of Supervisors that the provisions for the sick at the County Almshouse were inadequate, and that the rooms of the hospital were so overcrowded that they had to make arrangements with the managers of the [Brooklyn] City Hospital . . . to receive from the County Poorhouse a portion of the sick paupers."[50] At other times independent hospitals were funded to provide services that would maintain the social order: emergency services for the victims of industrial or streetcar accidents, ambulances in case of fire or other natural catastrophies, and shelter and aid to victims of crime, vagrants, alcoholics, and others who interfered with the city's life. During the winter months or during economic downswings these emergency services helped hold the community together. From its inception, city financing of such matters had been seen by public officials and those interested in limiting the scope of work in private facilities as an addendum to the financing of the public hospital.[51]

When public facilities became capable of absorbing all public dependents, Coler maintained that independent facilities had no more right to broad city support. He therefore set reimbursement rates at the level of maintenance costs for a hospital patient in Kings County, Bellevue, or some other municipal facility: "If private hospitals are to receive public assistance at all, payments should be made only at some uniform rate, approximately the same as the cost per capita of maintenance in the public institutions."[52] For Coler, the payment of funds to private facilities was wasteful, unless the city's own hospitals were overcrowded or overtaxed. "The city maintains its own hospitals, while at the same time subsidizing private institutions which compete with them," he noted.[53] During recent years, however,

> great improvements have been made in the city hospitals . . . While sometimes overcrowded, it frequently happens that the city hospitals are not filled to the limits . . . and it would seem as though the city should not deal with private hospitals except as subsidiary aids or adjuncts to the public institutions . . . It stands to reason that so long as there are vacant beds in the city hospitals, and the city is at the same time subsidizing private hospitals at a cost greater than the expense of caring for patients in its own institutions, a wrong is done to the taxpayers.[54]

Independent facilities were not at all in agreement with Coler's assessment of their status. From their point of view they functioned not to take advantage of public moneys but to prevent the dependence of indigent people on public services. At the very time when Coler began to view independent hospitals as wasteful, these hospitals saw themselves as providing charity services at great cost to themselves. They in fact expected more support from the city, particularly because they were feeling the increased financial burden of charity services just when they wanted to define their facilities as other than welfare insti-

Table 9. *Disposition of cases submitted by independent hospitals for reimbursement from the Department of Public Charities, 1902–1912*

	Accepted as proper charges		Rejected as proper charges		Total	
	N	%	N	%	N	%
1902	5,998	77.5	1,740	22.5	7,738	100
1903	7,017	81.2	1,624	18.8	8,641	100
1904	8,375	83.3	1,678	16.7	10,053	100
1905	9,106	83.4	1,815	16.6	10,921	100
1906	9,415	82	2,067	18	11,760	100
1907	9,897	84.2	1,863	15.8	11,760	100
1908	11,579	84.9	2,052	15.1	13,631	100
1909	11,954	83.7	2,319	16.3	14,273	100
1910	11,873	83.2	2,398	16.8	14,271	100
1911	11,743	78	3,307	22	15,050	100
1912	13,167	80.8	3,135	19.2	16,302	100

Note: In addition to patients with acute conditions, nursing mothers were also included in the city's reimbursement system. This table, then, includes dependent women who were nursing and, therefore, seen as appropriate for city care.

Source: New York City Department of Public Charities, *Annual Reports*, 1902–1912.

tutions. They considered that the growing plight of the urban and industrial poor was becoming almost intractable and demanded the increased attention and resources of the state, rather than the frail resources of private benevolence.

The city argued that charity should spend more on the poor – that, apart from reimbursement, charity should increase its responsibility to this class of people. Because decisions about reimbursement were ultimately made by the city, the hospitals were powerless in this discussion. The city decided to reject the claims made for poor persons who were not ambulance or emergency cases and who could have gone to the public hospitals. From 1902 to 1912, about 20 percent of cases submitted to the city for reimbursement were rejected (see Table 9), and of those cases rejected, between 67 and 80 percent were dismissed as nonemergency referrals. Because hospitals rarely presented cases that were financially inappropriate for city reimbursement, it is clear that trustees and administrators were now choosing cases to submit almost exclusively on the basis of economic class. Between 1902 and 1912 no more than 11 percent of rejections in any one year were a result of the patients' economic status (see Table 10).

1907						
No. of cases	1,289	201	148	225	0	1,863
% of total	69	11	8	12	0	100
1908						
No. of cases	1,434	173	155	290	0	2,052
% of total	70	8	8	14	0	100
1909						
No. of cases	1,536	201	196	386	0	2,319
% of total	66	9	8	17	0	100
1910						
No. of cases	1,593	251	169	485	0	2,498
% of total	64	10	7	19	0	100
1911						
No. of cases	2,056	264	285	696	6	3,307
% of total	62	8	9	21	0	100
1912						
No. of cases	2,039	204	242	643	7	3,135
% of total	65	7	8	21	0	101

[a] That is, nonresident, unknown at residence, referred to Kings County Hospital, or immigrant.
[b] Because of rounding, percentages do not always total to 100.
Source: New York City Department of Public Charities, Annual Reports, 1902–1912.

Table 10. *Reasons for rejection of reimbursement requests for hospital cases inspected in Brooklyn by the Department of Public Charities*

	Nonemergency	Able to pay	Discharged same day	Prearranged	Other[a]	Total
1902						
No. of cases	1,162	100	66	158	254	1,740
% of total	67	6	4	9	15	101[b]
1903						
No. of cases	1,325	86	48	136	29	1,624
% of total	82	5	3	8	2	100
1904						
No. of cases	1,415	82	40	130	11	1,678
% of total	84	5	2	8	1	100
1905						
No. of cases	1,347	128	237	93	10	1,815
% of total	74	7	13	5	1	100
1906						
No. of cases	1,552	173	161	181	0	2,067
% of total	75	8	8	9	0	100

By September 1901 it became clear that the effects of the reductions were to be felt mostly by the smaller, more precariously financed hospitals; the effects would be temporary on the larger, more stable institutions less directly dependent on public funds. "The results of the first year's work," reported Jesse Duryea, were that "seven hospitals [in Brooklyn and Queens] received more money than under the old system, while 18 received less." Duryea further noted that there was a drop of only $50,535 in the amount of public money distributed by the city government to the independent hospitals.[55] Significantly, the larger institutions were least affected by the drop in funds. Though the effects of the change could not be discounted, Duryea maintained that "the apprehension generally felt by hospital authorities that their funds were being cut off by the city was erroneous." Instead, the reforms only accentuated the fact "that there is a greater necessity for the existence of certain hospitals." Hospitals were being reimbursed for the work they did, and large, strong, useful institutions had little to fear from the reforms. Duryea recognized, however, that smaller hospitals or those without proper endowment might be adversely affected: "It is regrettable that some of the institutions most adversely affected by the new system are also the hospitals which were in the greatest financial embarrassment when the change was made."[56] Some hospitals went out of existence, others stopped accepting city patients, and the majority quickly adapted to the changed accounting system and standardized certain reporting procedures.

In spite of Coler's rhetoric of retrenchment, it became clear that the role of municipal government in funding health services was expanding rather than collapsing. Over the years, municipal funding for patients in most facilities increased. In Brooklyn, for example, hospitals submitted only 7,738 cases to the city for reimbursement in 1902, but by 1912 this number had increased to over 16,000. Though the city consistently rejected about 20 percent of all cases, the absolute number of cases rose steadily. The city paid for almost 6,000 patients in 1902 and 13,000 by 1912. This constituted a significant increase in reimbursement for a large institution with a large bed capacity. But this expansion came at the expense of the local trustees, who lost autonomy and control over reimbursement. Trustees could no longer accept any patients they wished but only those for whom they would be reimbursed by the city – that is, emergency and ambulance cases – or those who could pay for themselves. Smaller hospitals with limited bed capacity could not take advantage of the unlimited potential of per capita, per diem payment schemes, because they had no extra beds to fill with needy patients who would bring them city moneys. The change in payment mechanism accelerated the trustees' growing tendency to push administrators to pay close attention to the payment capabilities of patients, to initiate means tests, and to differentiate services according to class. It also forced trustees to relinquish whatever control over patient admissions they still maintained and to allow professionals greater control over the administration of the hospital. Generally, it commenced an ongoing process that forced small institutions to relate less to local community needs and more to the defined interests of central agencies far removed from local community pressures.

Community hospitals were not the only institutions offering health-related services to the growing number of poor immigrants in New York and Brooklyn's ethnic communities. Nor were they the only institutions that faced attacks from practitioners, the city, and the state during the Progressive era. The charity dispensaries, clinics that provided basic and specialty health services for large numbers of neighborhood residents, generally treated only those persons who needed "ambulatory" or outpatient services for endemic illnesses or chronic conditions. These dispensaries were largely unable to survive political and economic changes similar to those that wrought havoc with small charity hospitals.

6 Consolidating control over the small dispensary: the doctors, the city, and the state

As we have seen, the Progressive era brought major changes in the city's political and social arrangements. The demographic shifts, economic upheavals, and political reforms that undermined the cohesiveness of neighborhoods and their small hospitals also hurt the freestanding dispensaries and small walk-in clinics located throughout working-class neighborhoods. Like the small hospitals, dispensaries were nearly totally dependent upon the influence of local merchants and leaders to obtain city money for their survival. When power shifted from locally elected politicians to city officials and bureaucrats, and when the state comptroller's officials changed reimbursement regulations to favor large institutions, the freestanding dispensaries felt the pinch most severely.

The Progressive era's shift in the locus of decision making was accompanied by similar changes throughout the society. In commercial activities, large corporations replaced local businessmen. Everywhere, people tended to place greater and greater faith in large, impersonal, bureaucratic institutions, and to question the ability of smaller organizations to provide services. The locus of health-care services also shifted away from small-scale undertakings toward larger corporate institutions. Doctors' offices and the small dispensary were replaced by large hospitals with a wider base of financial support, more influential trustees, and a more extensive and sophisticated physical plant. Individual doctors moved to these larger institutions; dispensaries came to be regulated by the state; local merchant-trustees lost power to organized charity. The decline of the dispensary as a viable form of basic health-care delivery in the twentieth century reflects the move to corporate forms of health-care organization.

Late-nineteenth-century pressures on the dispensaries

In general, the nineteenth century witnessed the growth of two groups of dispensaries. Dispensaries of one type were affiliated with local hospitals as outpatient departments. The other group included small, unaffiliated, freestanding clinics sponsored by local merchants, grocers, pharmacists, and other neighborhood-based individuals. New York

146

alone had between seventy and eighty such facilities functioning during the 1890s.[1] These freestanding dispensaries, which were usually located in working-class neighborhoods, were organized in store fronts, tenements, and pharmacies; their services ranged from the provision of food and shelter to the provision of medical care. Like the small hospitals, these clinics grew up spontaneously in response to a felt need in the local community.

The local merchants and manufacturers who sponsored the dispensaries did so for a variety of reasons. A merchant in Manhattan's Lower East Side or Brooklyn's Greenpoint or Williamsburg section who joined with other area merchants to provide dispensary service to a rapidly expanding industrial work force could count on the respect of that community. Local pharmacists who organized a dispensary to function in conjunction with their drugstore could expect better business.[2] Unlike the trustees of large hospitals, who were often important in the *city's* social life and in large commercial enterprises, most of the trustees of small dispensaries were prominent only in their own neighborhoods.

Generally these local businessmen and civic leaders were marginally successful persons who could contribute little in the way of financial support to the clinics.[3] Their importance lay in their ability to lend legitimacy and local political clout to the institutions: The city was more likely to give funds to a facility sponsored by a reputable member of the community. Unfortunately for the dispensaries, the marginal positions of their trustees made them tremendously susceptible to the vagaries of economic depression and political rearrangements. In the nineteenth century, when local trustees had direct influence with the neighborhoods' aldermen and councilmen, who in turn had access to city money, dispensaries were fairly safe. But after the incorporation of Brooklyn into the larger city of New York in 1898, the locus of political power began to shift from local neighborhoods to City Hall in Manhattan and the State House in Albany. Dispensary trustees found themselves incapable of preventing crucial policy decisions that would effectively cripple their facilities.

In 1899 two acts taken by the city and state dealt severe blows to the city's clinics: Coler's efforts to limit funds for all small institutions; and the state legislature's imposition of strict regulations on dispensary practice through the Dispensary Law of 1899.

Doctors were among the first to call for the destruction of the dispensary. As a result of the conditions of medical practice and education during most of the nineteenth century, their relationship to the dispensaries was an ambiguous one. During the second half of the century, formal medical education rarely absorbed a great deal of time. Medical students often attended one of the numerous "proprietary" medical schools that turned out large numbers of graduates in a relatively short time. Sometimes organized for night instruction, sometimes catering to persons who had to work to support themselves, and generally without access to a hospital's wards, medical schools tended to provide little in the way of clinical experience for their students. The dispensary, therefore, was a place for training young doctors still attending or recently graduated from medical schools.

Because these schools were profit-making institutions that survived on the basis of their students' fees, they had a great incentive to admit large numbers of students and to make conditions for graduation relatively easy. The result was, of course, a highly crowded profession, especially for young doctors just beginning practice. Because a physician could rarely expect to establish a practice without a foothold in the neighborhood, a dispensary appointment was often a necessary step: Young practitioners would use the dispensaries in their neighborhoods to get clinical experience and to attract private patients.

More established community practitioners considered themselves to be in competition with the dispensary for patients, arguing that dispensaries catered to patients with marginal incomes who might otherwise use the services of a private doctor. "A great inroad into the practice of the profession is made by what I consider useless institutions in this city," declared Emmet Page, a private practitioner in Brooklyn, as early as 1888.[5] It was the "acknowledged abuse of the dispensaries by people who are able to employ a physician, yet are satisfied to apply for free treatment simply as a means of economy," that was most objectionable to Page. He called for the abolition of dispensaries "as a matter of protection to the profession."[6]

Page's article was part of a protracted discussion among private physicians caught in the vagaries of the changing medical marketplace. According to Page, the ability of private practitioners to control their future practice was threatened both by the population's growing acceptance of institutional care and by the eagerness of beginning practitioners to obtain dispensary appointments. "The younger members of the profession generally do the dispensary work," Page noted, "vainly hoping oftentimes to build up or start a practice."[7]

Yet the attitude of young practitioners toward the dispensaries was not always positive, because the dispensary made them dependent upon the institution's lay trustees for their positions. The clinics paid doctors little for their services and in some instances expected them to provide service out of a sense of noblesse oblige. Young physicians would therefore work hard for a reward that was a long time away – private patients. Some doctors resented the fact that the structure of the dispensary stirred up conflict between older physicians with marginal private practices and their younger colleagues, whom they saw as providing free care in the dispensaries.

Eventually the young doctors' resentments toward the dispensary led them to join with more established physicians in their call for a reduction in the number of dispensaries. "The paper of Dr. Page," the editors of the local medical journal observed, "contains much food for reflection." The editors urged "vigorous action" to reduce the number of dispensaries "and to change the practice in those that remain."[8] A decrease in the number of dispensaries and a limitation in patient access would lessen the importance of these facilities and lower their impact on private practice. Doctors called for regulations that would force clinics to serve only the "truly" indigent, so that the legitimate needs of education for younger members would be met and private practices would also be protected.

By the end of the century, the structure of medical practice changed in ways that also made doctors less dependent on the dispensary. First, doctors increasingly sought to establish practices in wealthier neighborhoods at some distance from the dispensaries. Second, medical education became more specialized and began to be organized around clinics and hospitals, thereby providing students with more clinical experience. Also, as was discussed in Chapter 4, doctors were rapidly gaining access to hospital appointments. These additional options enabled them to refuse dispensary appointments. By turning to the hospital for their education, professional advancement, and clinical training, physicians freed themselves of control by the trustees of the dispensaries.[9]

The waning interest of physicians in dispensary practice was reflected in their growing absenteeism. As early as 1881, the Bushwick and East Brooklyn Dispensary, a small institution in the northern working-class section of the city, reported that "changes in the Medical and Surgical staff have not been infrequent."[10] But by the early 1890s, such statements took on a new and added significance. At the Central Dispensary, the head of the medical staff "regretted" the "irregularity in attendance" of two members of his staff.[11] At the Eastern District Dispensary, the president, George Fisher, reported that among a number of physicians "there has been a degree of absenteeism which is inconsistent with the interests of our patients and the institution."[12]

Absenteeism was reflective of a larger movement against the dispensaries. By the early 1890s a serious and far-reaching movement was under way to limit what was commonly called the "Dispensary Abuse," the abuse of free services by those who could afford to pay private physicians. Most practitioners agreed that the number of and access to dispensaries had to be limited in some way in order to control the perceived effect on private practice. To discourage the use of these institutions by nonindigent persons, doctors invoked moral, legal, and professional sanctions. Louis F. Criado, a Brooklyn physician, read a paper before the Kings County Medical Association in 1893 that enumerated a series of "necessary" dispensary reforms. He argued that the dispensary should be solely a "welfare" institution and that fines should be imposed on nonindigent persons who used the facility. He also suggested that "at the entrance hall and in every dispensary room occupied by physicians, a large placard should be displayed in a conspicuous place making it known that the institution is intended for the care of the destitute poor *only*."[13] Furthermore, Criado declared, dispensary physicians should vow never to treat patients whom they considered capable of paying a private doctor.

Private and dispensary physicians alike took up the cry to limit the use of the dispensary only to those unable to pay private doctors. At the Eastern District Dispensary, Dr. Samuel Brown declared his personal decision to stop treating patients he deemed able to pay for private services. "I am treating nothing but the worthy poor who apply to my clinic for treatment," he announced to the trustees in 1891. He reported that his recently adopted criteria for judging the proper recipients of his services made him "able to say that every patient I prescribe for is unable to obtain a doctor's services. In this way I protect the institution and at the same time do justice to my outside fellow practitioners, whose patients find their way into my clinic daily."[14] The *Brooklyn Medical Journal* noted this physician's declaration and added that if "equal care were taken in all the dispensaries, much of the criticism which has justly been made upon these institutions . . . would be no longer applicable."[15] Doctors hoped, in the early 1890s, that they could solve their own problems.

Explicit policies helped to reorganize dispensaries, but more subtle factors were also at work. Because physicians were primarily committed to private practice, they chose to neglect their commitment to dispensaries when demand for private services was high. "This epidemic [of influenza] was a sore tax upon the powers of endurance of the members of the staff," reported the medical secretary of one dispensary in 1890. The epidemic had given doctors "all they could do in their private practice" and caused widespread absenteeism at the dispensary.[16]

Although dispensary managers identified private practice as a major reason for absenteeism among doctors, they also recognized that the lack of appropriate equipment and supplies lowered doctors' commitment to dispensaries. It was difficult to provide adequate care in poorly equipped, understaffed places. Managers recognized "that the doctors would take more interest in their work, and the clinics would be better attended, if our quarters were more commodious."[17]

Doctors' objections to the dispensary intensified during the Depression of the 1890s, as they witnessed the growing dependence of people on inexpensive dispensary services. Private practitioners feared that patients would come to accept clinics as a viable alternative to the private office. In 1894 the Central Dispensary noted that "hard times" were responsible for the large increase in the number of patients. The facility serviced over 4,000 more patients than it had in the year before. At the same time, private doctors complained of *decreasing* patient demand. Given the dispensaries' rapid and obvious increase in patients, it was only logical for private practitioners to conclude that the dispensaries' expansion was in part accomplished at the practitioners' expense.[18]

Though doctors were united in their call for the abolition of the dispensary, they recognized their own internal differences and their inability to effect the demise of the dispensary. Because neither the American Medical Association nor the local medical society was as yet a powerful force, doctors lacked a single organization to represent their common interests. It was also a fact that, despite their agreement on the need to limit dispensaries, the younger physicians were still partly dependent upon them. Finally, doctors might share certain interests, but they essentially saw themselves as competitors in a crowded market.

Therefore, whereas earlier critics had called for doctors to solve the dispensary-abuse issue themselves, the 1890s saw the growing acceptance of external forms of regulatory activity as a viable means of controlling them. In their medical journals, doctors began to press for state and city regulation as a way to solve the abuse problem. The *Brooklyn Medical Journal*, for instance, noted that it was, "perhaps, rather Utopian" to assume "that the profession has it in its own power to correct [the] abuses and confine the privileges of those institutions to those for whom they were intended."[19] Government, in conjunction with the profession itself, was now called upon to enter into dispensary regulation.

The redistribution of city funds and the Dispensary Law of 1899

City government dealt the first staggering blow to the dispensaries by limiting the funds available to them. With the incorporation of Brooklyn into the City of New York and the reorganization of governmental activities, the locus of power shifted from Brooklyn and the local city council to New York and the comptroller's office in lower Manhattan. Dispensary trustees quickly lost their ability to obtain municipal funds. Comptroller Coler, elected by the city at large, was not dependent upon the goodwill of locally based grocers, manufacturers, and pharmacists in the city's poorer neighborhoods and could make decisions with little attention to the particular interests of a neighborhood.

A year after entering the comptroller's office, Coler integrated a policy of substantial reductions in dispensary appropriations into his general reform of public charity. City funds were reserved, he explained, for larger charity organizations that could show they were doing work for which the city was responsible. The city held that large facilities providing housing and inpatient services were clearly fulfilling a needed service for the destitute. Those institutions which catered to outpatients and provided "outdoor" relief were considered to be providing services to persons not uniformly without means and, therefore, not appropriate as city charges.[20] "Many [organizational] recipients of public funds devote themselves exclusively to outdoor relief," noted Coler, "and . . . however proper these may be as the [objects] of private benevolence, they are extremely improper objects of the public bounty." Coler suggested that the "immediate and permanent discontinuance of [public] appropriations to all such societies and institutions will correct one of the gravest abuses of the present system."[21]

Coler instituted a phased withdrawal of funds available to small dispensaries. The city adopted a rule by which dispensaries would never receive more than 50 percent of the amount collected from private sources. Although large charity institutions could expect to maintain a substantial income from city coffers, small facilities could not. No dispensary could expect to continue operations if it lacked a wide base of support from wealthy philanthropists or societies.[22]

The new regulations "wiped out of existence a number of dispensaries of mushroom growth which depended exclusively upon city money for support," Coler observed early in the century.[23] These small unaffiliated dispensaries, often located in the industrial working-class neighborhoods in the northeast section of Brooklyn, clearly felt the crunch of the new city policy. The Bushwick and East Brooklyn Dispensary, for instance, had for many years run on an income of $1,500 derived from municipal sources. But in 1901 its president noted that "the Management has practically no subscription list at all" – a lack which meant that the donation from the city would be small. "The city's appropriation to us was unprecedentedly small and not what it would seem we were fairly entitled to," he complained.[24] Subsequent years were increasingly precarious, and by 1906 the city subsidy was only $241. "We are doing work that the city ought to pay for," declared the president of the organization in 1911. "But we receive only about $250 a year from it."[25]

The professional opposition of local doctors and the city's financial retrenchment were but two prongs of the attack on dispensaries. In the mid-1890s the state, the largest of the units involved in charity regulation, began an investigation, and the resulting bill, finally passed in 1899, dealt the final death blow to the small dispensaries. Prompted by pressure from medical societies, hospitals, and private physicians, the State Board of Charities assigned a prominent physician, Stephen Smith, and two laymen, Enoch Stoddard and Tunis Bergen, to an investigating committee. It was clear that anything the state might do to cut the number of and access to the dispensary would satisfy private practitioners, and anything that raised standards and the quality of service would be readily supported by hospital-based specialists and physicians. When the report was issued, and ultimately, the bill passed, the medical profession rejoiced. The *Brooklyn Medical Journal* editorialized that the bill was "an excellent one" that should have "the hearty support of the medical profession."[26]

The report that led to the legislative action summarized the numerous problems plaguing the health-care system as a whole. The report maintained that, in earlier times, the few dispensaries that existed posed no threat to the practice of community doctors, who considered dispensaries part of a system of medical relief that served "only the sick poor . . . unable to pay for either advice or medicine." Doctors also knew that the number of poor using these services was relatively limited before the massive immigration to New York and the growth of an industrial economy. It was only when dispensaries grew and diversified their functions, and began to attract more patients, that doctors began to think of the dispensaries as encroaching upon their territory.[27]

The investigators who reported on the state of the dispensaries considered that there were few alternatives to legislative action that could possibly correct the numerous abuses plaguing these facilities. "There is no evidence that the system has within its own organization any force active or latent, that will finally reform its operations," the investigators noted. "The only power that can deal adequately with the dispensary is the body which created it, the Legislature." Furthermore, "the evils of our dispensary system have reached such a magnitude that the Legislature cannot long delay action." Accepting the need for state control and regulation of the dispensaries, the report said that necessary supervision could only come from the State Board of Charities, which had recently been charged by the legislature and the state constitution with the responsibility for visiting and inspecting "all institutions, whether State, county, municipal, incorporated or not incorporated which are of a charitable, eleemosynary, correctional or reformatory character." The report concluded that this broad constitutional mandate made it "apparent that the whole field of reform of medical charities comes within the immediate jurisdiction of the State Board of Charities."[28] Thus dispensaries, as charity or "welfare" organizations, were an appropriate place for state regulation.

The role of the state in the supervision of the various charities had been expanding for a number of years before the report was issued. In the 1890s the legislature became involved in protecting healthy dependent children, and empowered the board to certify for incorporation all institutions in the state that proposed to maintain "nursing children or others under the age of twelve."[29] As the success of this venture became known, the state moved to increase its involvement in the regulation of dispensaries and other charities as well, primarily in order to promote efficiency in their management.

The state committee quickly remarked that "it is not difficult to indicate some of the more important powers which should be conferred . . . to relieve the dispensaries of the evils which result from injurious management." The committee recommended that the Board of Charities have the power to prevent the establishment of unnecessary new dispensaries or those that might be started by unqualified individuals; to compel dispensaries to update and improve the services for their patients; and to require that dispensaries "adopt and maintain a uniform system of records" that would provide information on the "social condition of each applicant, [and] the finances of the institution," and "maintain an investigation of the worthiness of each applicant for the relief sought."[30]

The medical profession enthusiastically endorsed the legislation drafted as a result of the committee's report. The agitation of the profession, it was recognized, "resulted in an appeal to the legislature, to which body reformers always turn when in their opinion a widespread error exists which needs to be vigorously combatted."[31]

As with any reform, support for and opposition to the bill came from several sources, all of which had different concerns. When the bill was first presented in 1897 it failed to pass. Homeopaths and other schools of physicians objected that "only one school [of medicine] was represented" on the Board of Charities, which was empowered to oversee the regulatory activities. Some critics argued that the financial plight of the physicians resulted from "overcrowding of the medical profession" and that dispensary abuse was a false issue. "The true remedy [is] to reduce the number of doctors," remarked one medical journal. Some lay persons considered the bill an attempt by physicians "to deprive the public of medical help at reasonable rates and thus drive them into their offices and extort exorbitant fees."[32]

But the most serious objections came from some of the powerful dispensaries themselves. Administrators of large hospital-based dispensaries, sensing that the bill might be used to allow the state to interfere with the internal workings of their institutions, lobbied hard against the first bills in 1897 and 1898. Only when it was made clear that the bill was specifically designed to attack freestanding dispensaries, not hospital outpatient departments, did the large institutions drop their opposition.[33]

The final Dispensary Law of 1899 was aimed at correcting a broad set of abuses most obvious in the smaller dispensaries. On October 11, 1899, just ten days after the Dispensary Law went into effect, the State Board of Charities enacted a series of "Rules and Regulations." The first of these rules was intended to limit access to the dispensaries; it required that each dispensary post a public notice in a "conspicuous place" threatening imprisonment of nonindigent patients who tried to use the facility.[34] The next few rules concerned the quality and kinds of services to be dispensed at these facilities. They required that a matron be present for gynecological exams, and that anyone with a contagious disease be excluded from the facility. No longer could religious instruction be required of patients. A licensed apothecary or a graduate of an incorporated medical college had to be present for the disbursement of drugs, and separate seating arrangements had to be provided for men and women in the waiting room. While these rules raised the standards of care in dispensaries, they simultaneously defined these institutions as a welfare service by restricting them to the care of the "truly" indigent.

The rules imposed by the Board of Charities initially had an uneven effect. In 1901 the journal *Charities* reported that a third of the dispensaries in New York City had not posted the public notice threatening imprisonment for nonindigent patients. Other dispensaries failed to provide restrictions on contagious-disease cases. The rules may have been designed to be "so stringent that they would effectually remedy the evils for which the law was enacted," but many dispensary managers in New York were bypassing them.[35] There was also initial concern and confusion about the effectiveness of the law in Brooklyn. Although the local medical journal did report that one of Brooklyn's largest dispensaries showed a significant decrease in the number of applicants accepted by dispensary authorities, other institutions were suspected of lax regulation of patients.[36]

The managers of the stabler hospital-affiliated dispensaries had fewer objections to the law than had been expected. Although some acknowledged an unfortunate decline in patient loads because of the "operation of the dispensary law," others judged there were benefits as well. The "mere knowledge of the existence of the law and its requirements has probably deterred many from making application. . . . It cannot be avoided, after a single years [sic] experience that its enactment was legislation in the right direction and gives promise of great benefit." The bill was welcomed by those who supported efforts to label the dispensary a "welfare" institution for the "indigent poor only."[37]

By 1905 most acknowledged that the law had caused significant change in at least some dispensary practices. There was general agreement that the law promoted internal reorganization. William H. Buck, in a 1905 article in *Charities*, noted that important reforms had occurred in the dispensaries' cleanliness, care, and administration. In a survey of 119 dispensaries in New York State in 1905, Buck found significant changes in administrative procedures: 118 had a registrar, 114 took and preserved records, all issued pass cards, and 110 had the appropriate penalty printed on the pass cards. Service seemed to meet certain minimum standards of quality: 116 dispensaries examined all applicants, and 51 provided "thorough" examinations. One hundred seventeen facilities had matrons present; 115 were clean and orderly; and all dispensaries excluded contagious diseases. Buck concluded, however, that although the law furthered the administrative and hygienic reform of many facilities, it did little to improve the control of dispensary abuse: So-called well-to-do patients continued to use the dispensary.[38]

The problem was how to define "well-to-do." During the Depression of the 1890s many of the city's poor needed direct and constant aid from organized charity. Differentiating among the poor was seen as an inexact and perilous enterprise, particularly during a period of great need.[39] Only the Brooklyn Association for Improving the Conditions of the Poor, whose "bureau of investigation [had] been so tested and perfected by years of experience," felt it could make "without serious delay or friction . . . the required discrimination" between worthy and unworthy individuals.[40] For small dispensaries and individuals with more humility such fine discriminations were problematic at best. All that managers could do was entreat their staff to "be vigilant, and reject all unworthy applicants."[41]

Dispensary managers and clinicians had difficulty distinguishing between medical and social criteria for admissions to their institutions. No one had a really effective way of separating medical need from its social manifestations. In 1898 dispensary managers formed an organization to develop such criteria and to "ascertain the extent of the evil," as it was called. But attempts to "devise methods for [the evil's] diminution, and, if possible, its abatement" failed to result in any lasting and effective means of deciding which patients were medically needy and which needed care, shelter, and food.[42] In the absence of such criteria all dispensaries endeavored to "guard against treating [abusers] as far as possible." But most agreed with the Central Throat Hospital that it "is surely better to benefit a few unworthy imposters than that one deserving poor person should suffer from want of proper medical aid."[43]

The Dispensary Law had important, although uneven, effects upon the organization of the health institutions in New York and Brooklyn. It lent the authority of the state to a movement to reorganize the internal administration of the dispensary and to activate external state regulation of health facilities. But the Dispensary Law barely satisfied the concerns of those who mobilized professional support for the law. By 1905 "there was . . . good evidence that the primary purpose for which the law was created," namely, that of guaranteeing a stable clientele to doctors in private practice, was not being accomplished. There was a "widespread feeling among practitioners that they [were still] deprived of reasonable fees by the multiplicity of free services." This perception of the threat posed by dispensaries to private doctors would continue until the pressure of competition from hospital-affiliated outpatient departments, the many dispensaries, and emergency rooms combined with reduced support from the city government to put an end to the dispensary system itself.[44] Ultimately, private practice as well as small dispensaries would give way to large corporate forms of medical-care delivery.

The Brooklyn City Dispensary

The Brooklyn City Dispensary, one of the city's freestanding clinics, exemplified the plight of many small institutions. Begun in the 1880s as a charitable enterprise supported by such prestigious Brooklynites as Henry E. Pierrepont and Charles Adams, this dispensary faced tremendous problems at the end of the nineteenth century. City and state attempts to regulate the dispensaries and the declining interest of doctors in this institution proved fatal. It averted closure for a number of years – first as a health clinic and then as a dental clinic – but finally succumbed to financial pressures late in the Progressive era and closed entirely.

As late as 1897, the medical director and trustees at the Brooklyn City Dispensary noted that their patient rolls were continuing to grow.[45] Between 1895 and 1896, the Depression and the lack of alternative health services in poor neighborhoods pressed over 300 additional working-class patients into this dispensary. In 1895 nearly 18,500 persons were treated; in 1896 the figure was over 18,800. Of these people, over half were new cases in each of the years.[46]

The cost of running this institution was modest, amounting to less than 15 cents per case. In 1897 the trustees of the Brooklyn City Dispensary spent a mere $2,323, of which $1,440 paid the salaries of the pharmacist, the maintenance staff, and the registrar. Medical supplies cost only $533 and fuel $130. Eighty-three percent of the income for this institution came from the City of Brooklyn in the form of a $1,500 grant for servicing the city's poor and $800 from the city's excise fund. Only $532 came from donations or legacies.[47]

By the end of the decade, the medical staff was increasingly uninterested in the dispensary and in support of a growing movement to regulate this and other facilities. From June of 1896 until the early 1900s the poor attendance and tardiness of the medical staff was a chronic problem for the trustees. At first, the trustees' committees issued mild reprimands and asked the "medical director to advise the absentees to be more considerate of the patients."[48] But the problem of absenteeism became increasingly severe. The "attendance of the staff has been very irregular and unsatisfactory," remarked one trustee in October of 1896. "Dr. Night has been away for two months without a substitute and has not been heard from. Dr. Commbs left a substitute for one week and was gone two months."[49] By December of 1896, the president observed that "the Medical staff had been so irregular in its attendance that he and the medical director devised a form to be filled out by the doctors applying hereafter for appointment."[50] The form included a summary of an article in the dispensary by-laws that said, in part: "No physician shall absent himself from duty without the consent of the visiting committee . . . Any physician who shall absent himself from duty . . . four times in succession . . . without being excused, shall be reported."[51] With few doctors present and an increased number of patients, the dispensary was continually over-crowded. The doctors are "still tardy . . . the reception room crowded and the air very bad," noted a trustee in early 1897.[52] By December the visiting committee "found the backroom full of patients and bad odors," with few doctors around.[53]

Because many community practitioners had moved to new areas of the city and established practices where hospital appointments were easy to attain, trustees found it difficult to replace their absentee physician staff. In April 1899, the "Committee on Staff reported that better attendance could not be pushed . . . since there were no applications" for staff positions from local doctors.[54] By 1902 there "was much dissention as to absences of doctors," but trustees could do little about it.[55] Doctors also remained associated with the dispensary for shorter periods of time. Of the nineteen physicians who served between 1893 and 1903, only two worked there five years or more. Five stayed on staff for eighteen to twenty-four months, two stayed from twelve to thirteen months, and five stayed from one to eleven months. This rapid turnover continued into the early years of the twentieth century.[56]

Toward the end of the century the Brooklyn City Dispensary was secure in its dependence on municipal funds. Trustees kept a constant watch over Brooklyn City Hall to make sure that appropriations for the dispensary would be included in the budget. When, in 1896, the trustees' "Excise Committee" reported that the usual appropriation for the institutions had been omitted in the city's annual budget, it took little time for the trustees to get in touch with their local representative to confirm that this was merely an oversight that would be corrected after the first of the year.[57] With power for such decisions residing in the hands of local officials, trustees felt fairly confident that the city would respond to their demands and interests.

By 1899, however, Brooklyn was incorporated into the City of New York and financial power had shifted to Manhattan, so that city funds were less accessible. In October 1898 one trustee reported that the $800 usually appropriated to the dispensary from the municipal government's excise fund (tax money derived from sales of liquor, bars, and other businesses that the mores of the time found questionable) would not be available after January 1, 1899, the date Brooklyn and Manhattan merged. Judging that they could do little to influence the actions of city officials in Manhattan, the trustees recommended that "a committee be formed to find some new sources of revenue to take the place of the old income."[58] Even the most prestigious of the trustees had little power. When one trustee went to see the comptroller of

New York City "with the view of getting money to take the place of the $800 formerly received," he was informed that special treatment could not be shown to Brooklyn's dispensaries. After all, though Brooklyn's dispensaries had been given city excise appropriations, the Manhattan facilities had not.[59] The comptroller made a vague promise that some funds would be available in the future. Not only were the dispensaries cut off from excise money, but the per capita reimbursement scheme that replaced the older $1,500 flat grant left dispensaries in financial disorder. "It is possible that some additional revenues may be obtained from the City in the future," lamented one frustrated trustee, "but . . . it would be necessary to show a need for an increase" in reimbursement.[60]

By January 1900 the trustees of Brooklyn City Dispensary appointed a committee "to find out where we stand financially . . . so that the Board can act understandingly" in the future.[61] In February the finance committee reported "that the money to be received from the city would be $398.12, a sum totally inadequate for the expenses of the institution."[62] In October the president of the trustees reported that his attempts "to obtain larger appropriations from the city through the Comptroller" had been fruitless and that another committee was appointed "to see what could be done."[63] In November a committee reported that next year's appropriation would be only $259.[64] Things were getting worse. For the first time in over a decade, the dispensary was running at a deficit of over $600.[65]

At this time, with the change in the city comptroller's office already posing a large problem, the state also sought to change its dispensary practices. In 1897, when the first dispensary bill was put before the legislature, the trustees of the various dispensaries were able to exert enough pressure to kill it. But another bill was soon presented, after prompting from the state's medical societies. In February 1898, at Brooklyn City Dispensary, a "special meeting [of the Board] was called . . . to take action against the bill." The board appointed a committee to meet with other dispensary representatives to discuss means of stopping passage. "It was unanimously voted that the officers . . . attend [a meeting] to be held at the Hotel Manhattan . . . with full discretionary powers," reported the secretary of the board.[66] The very next week, the board moved that two representatives "go before the legislative committee to protest against the [bill's] passage . . . and that a letter to this same effect be sent to our Representative at Albany."[67] In April the board joined with other local dispensary representatives to work toward "protecting such institutions from unjust attacks through the Legislature."[63]

The trustees at the City Dispensary recognized that it was only a matter of time before some form of the Dispensary Bill was passed. When "a communication from the State Board of Charities" was received, "asking for suggestions as to the licensing and regulation of dispensaries," the board made few suggestions and tried to ignore the possibility of means tests, inspections, and other forms of regulation.[69] In February 1900, after the Dispensary Bill was passed, the trustees noted the effects of the new regulations. One commented that there was already a "small falling off in the number of patients since the new arrangements were inaugurated by the State Board of Charities." The future of the dispensary seemed bleak.[70]

To forestall an impending financial crisis, the dispensary corporation sold property, moved to a cheaper location, and began charging patients for services previously provided without charge. The dispensary board initially took money from the dispensary's reserve fund in the Dime Savings Bank and transferred it to the general fund, thereby depleting the Dispensary's cash reserves to a mere $376.[71] Although trustees knew that more cash would be needed for the institution to survive and that transfers were a long-term threat to its financial stability, they found few alternatives that did not threaten the dispensary's viability. In April 1900 the money derived from the sale of a piece of dispensary property was diverted from an interest-earning investment to the fund "used to meet current expenses."[72] Having sold property that represented a goodly portion of the dispensary's endowment, some trustees next sought to tax themselves more heavily. Also in April, the trustees engaged in a "lengthy discussion" about an amendment to the bylaws that would force "each trustee [to] contribute annually the sum of ten dollars for the uses of the dispensary." Twelve trustees rejected this recommendation, and only three favored it. The issue was really whether trustees should donate their money freely rather than be taxed. After the measure was rejected, one trustee offered a voluntary measure that would accomplish the same thing: He moved that "the roll be called and each trustee be called on to say what he would do to help meet the deficiency."[73]

In October the board's president wrote a letter stating that the projected deficit for the dispensary would be about "$600 in spite of the subscription raised." The board then had another lengthy discussion, in which it was decided that a "charge of 10 cents for every prescription" would be made to patients using the facility.[74] Although such a charge contradicted what the trustees saw as the charitable purpose of the facility, the board was forced to acknowledge that it was necessary for the institution's survival. Exceptions could be made for the "especially poor," but this would require a judgment and evaluation by the institution's director.[75]

By December a small study revealed that $18.25 had been earned in a period of eight days from such charges and that over $900 could be collected in a year's time. By 1901 a charge of 5 cents was instituted for all bottles used when filling a prescription. By 1904 the practice was accepted, and the trustees decided that "no change in its present plan of charging for prescriptions" should be made.[76]

Ironically, the movement to charge patients eventually led to a loss of city funds and a worse crisis. The institution was designated by the state as a charity, and as such, it was intended to serve the poor and only the poor. By instituting charges, the trustees were acknowledging that not all of the dispensary's patients were indigent. The state would see this admission as evidence that the dispensary was not a "welfare" institution worthy of public money. In their attempt to save the dispensary by charging patients a small fee, the trustees were actually forgoing one of their most important sources of funds – public money.

The turn away from charity came about only after other attempts to save the dispensary had failed. In 1903 the trustees tried to gain stability by merging with Brooklyn Hospital, a larger institution. This plan fell through when it became apparent that the hospital had no interest in maintaining the dispensary as an identifiable entity, because it had its own outpatient departments and specialized clinics.[77] The dispensary turned instead to advertising and was able thereby to effect a modest but temporary increase in its clients.[78]

By the middle years of the Progressive era, it was clear that the Brooklyn City Dispensary's days were numbered. Services had contracted, doctors' services were declining, and working-class patients were beginning to seek services through the hospital's growing outpatient departments. The endowment of the facility was quickly eroded, and by 1920 the facility stopped providing medical services altogether. It became a modestly sized dental clinic.[79]

By the time of its demise, the dispensary became identified solely with what is today referred to as "welfare medicine." Identification cards, signs, and popular propaganda served to alert people to the degradation and stigmatization that awaited them in underfinanced, understaffed, small, crowded institutions. By the 1920s few unaffiliated, freestanding dispensaries continued in existence. The hospital-affiliated dispensaries that survived took on the less objectionable title "outpatient department," although to this day they still serve those unable to pay a private physician. Although change in these nineteenth-century facilities had been necessary, the intervention of the state, the city, and professional groups destroyed an important service once available to the working class. Furthermore, the concentration of resources in large facilities served to deemphasize the importance of outpatient services while accentuating the medical profession's orientation toward inpatient, high-technology medicine.

7   The battle for Morningside Heights:
power and politics in the
boardroom of New York Hospital

New York and Brooklyn community hospitals and dispensaries were organized and run by local church groups, merchants, and other organizations and leaders. These sponsors lent to their institutions the ethnic or religious flavor that made the services unique. Rarely, if ever, were the trustees and governors important on the regional, state, or national level. When the forces of industrial and economic change, commercial development, or demographic reorganization and political upheaval altered the relationships and neighborhoods in which these institutions were located, the hospitals found themselves subjected to pressures well beyond their control. In the face of these growing pressures, smaller institutions sometimes moved away or reorganized, or perhaps went out of existence.

For some Manhattan hospitals, the story was different. Some hospitals were larger, had more political power, and were more secure financially. Their lay governors and trustees often came from older and more prominent New York families who controlled and owned significant portions of the city and provided access to benefactors, legacies, and landholdings. Given the enormous financial and political resources of these institutions and their trustees, it is not surprising to find that when they came into conflict with the forces of urbanization and capitalist development that seriously disrupted smaller facilities, the outcomes were substantially different. Although larger hospitals and institutions were often pressured to move by realtors, they generally had more control over where they moved and how they affected neighborhoods than did community hospitals. Some were able, for example, to see that power was not shifted from the city's Protestant elites to a new class of entrepreneurs of lower social standing.

A case in point is the experience of the governors of the Society of New York Hospital, one of the city's largest and oldest charity institutions. In the 1880s, as the city's immigrant neighborhoods spread uptown, the hospital's landholdings in the uptown regions of Manhattan became the focus of a dramatic battle for control. In the area called Morningside Heights, the hospital held about thirty-five acres of land between 110th Street and 120th Street on the West Side of the city. Real estate developers, interested in extending to the west the building boom then going on in Harlem, sought to gain control over this land, on which sat the hospital's Bloomingdale Insane Asylum. The governors of the hospital, interested first in saving their asylum and second in directing the future development of the community, fought a long battle to maintain control over the neighborhood. Because the governors were able to exert considerable political pressure, the battle lasted a number of years.

Under intense pressure from Tammany Hall, the state senate and assembly, major real estate speculators, and nearly all of the city's newspapers, the hospital's governors were forced to move their asylum off the land in the late 1880s and early 1890s. But they relinquished the land in ways which guaranteed that the neighborhood would be maintained largely as a bastion of middle- and upper-class Protestant respectability within a city that was being inundated by Catholic and Jewish working-class groups. In the years between 1889 and 1902 the hospital's governors sold large tracts of its holdings to Columbia and Barnard College, the city's elite Protestant-led educational institutions. Scattered blocks and lots were sold to private developers with the proviso that only residences for the wealthy would be built. In this way, the hospital played an important role in shaping the social makeup and class characteristics of a significant neighborhood long after the hospital had relinquished formal control over the area.

The story of the battle over Morningside Heights illustrates the importance of the hospital trustees in the city's social life. During this period centralized governmental agencies had no significant control over the planning process.[1] At a time when New York's political life and neighborhoods were being overwhelmed by the massive immigration of Eastern and Southern Europeans, Irish and Italian Catholics, and Jews, the battle for control of land use was fought by older Protestant merchants and bankers through places like the boardroom of New York Hospital.

Property and hospital financing during the late nineteenth century

New York Hospital's involvement in the city's real estate market began in 1866, just after the Civil War. The hospital came out of the war in debt, and its governors proposed a plan that would "relieve this charitable corporation from present and prospective pecuniary embarrassment" through real estate development and investment.[2] The report proposed that the hospital move from its location in the downtown area near City Hall to a less expensive piece of land farther uptown near Union Square. The original hospital site at City Hall could then be sold or rented for long-term financial rewards. "A very general conviction exists that the New York Hospital could place itself out of debt, and be supplied with ample means for greatly extended usefulness . . . by sale or lease of the hospital grounds," a committee of the governors reported in 1866. "The Hospital lands have become very valuable for commercial purposes," and the hospital could find land farther uptown "in some other locality."[3]

In the eyes of the governors, the use of land to produce income was an important and necessary departure from the traditional manner by which charities supported themselves. "The conviction is that not only of the thoughtless multitudes that such a move is necessary, but also of benevolent thoughtful men, who sympathize with the objects of the institution, and are not unaware of the apparent obstacles in the way of such a radical step," they noted.[4] By the end of the Civil War the governors of New York Hospital controlled the land upon which the hospital then sat at Broadway and Church streets in lower Manhattan; a few lots, 25 feet by 100 feet, on Ninth Avenue and Twenty-ninth Street; and large tracts of land at Morningside Heights, then a rural area of Manhattan, where Bloomingdale, the hospital's mental asylum, was located.[5]

During the last third of the century, the New York Hospital successfully tied its future to the vagaries of the city real estate markets. In 1866 the hospital received only $61 per year in income from property and rents. By 1886, two decades later, the institution received over $150,000 per year, more than a third of its annual income, from rents on its various properties. By the end of the century, the hospital's land in the downtown area was assessed at over $2.67 million and large tracts of land in the Twelfth Ward in the uptown section were valued at over $1.67 million. In all, the hospital controlled land in New York City and Westchester valued at over $5.5 million.[6]

Whereas the downtown property at City Hall and Ninth Avenue was important as a source of income for the hospital, the uptown land at Morningside Heights was the site of the hospital's asylum. Bloomingdale had been established in 1821 in what was then the rural township of Bloomingdale, New York. Cut off from the center of New York City by four miles of unleveled land and poor transportation and communication, Bloomingdale was considered, in the early nineteenth century, ideally isolated and rural for an asylum. The largely wooded area rested on a high bluff overlooking the Hudson River, with New Jersey's Palisades to the west and then bucolic Harlem on the east.

The rapid uptown growth of New York began to impinge upon this tract of land, however, by the second half of the century. When the city bought land to build Central Park in 1858, land values in adjacent areas on the East and West sides improved. The Third Avenue Elevated Railroad was opened to 129th Street in 1878. In 1880 the Second Avenue El opened up the East Side and the Ninth Avenue El opened the West Side.[7] By the early 1880s land values on the East Side were skyrocketing, and the West Side was steadily expanding uptown. As millions of immigrants arrived in New York, and as transportation improved and the economy exploded, there was steady pressure to develop housing for both the wealthy and the poor in previously inaccessible areas of the city.

The rapid growth of the city profoundly affected the hospital's landholdings at Morningside Heights. These thirty-five acres of property between 110th and 120th streets were among the most beautiful in the city and became prime real estate as the building boom of the 1880s spread from the East Side westward into Central Harlem as well as up the West Side. The construction of Riverside Park beginning in 1877 and of Morningside Park in 1868 made the previously inaccessible Bloomingdale Asylum land extremely valuable for residential sites.[8] The Ninth Avenue El, with its stop at 116th Street and Eighth Avenue, allowed for the development of either an economically mixed or a working-class neighborhood.

It was apparent that the West Side would be a major focus for development in the 1880s. But the social and class characteristics of the West Side were still undetermined. The avenues along the Hudson River and Central Park, most agreed, would be residences for the wealthy. Riverside Drive and Central Park West were to be lined with mansions or fancy apartment buildings like the Dakota, which was planned at Seventy-second Street in 1880. The streets and avenues between the Hudson River and the various parks were still to be divided. Whereas some predicted that the upper West Side would house only the wealthy, others recognized that the elevated made the area appropriate for working-class groups as well. There were those who predicted that Ninth and Tenth avenues (renamed Columbus and Amsterdam avenues in 1880) would become a tenement district of Irish and blacks "like the . . . blocks south of West Fifty-Ninth Street."[9] By the early 1880s real estate speculators interested in extending Harlem and the West Side eyed eagerly all available land west of Broadway. It seemed inevitable that a boom in land values would eventually overtake the neighborhood.

In Morningside Heights, the presence of the hospital's asylum, housing 250 mental patients, blocked development and severely depressed the value of landholdings. "There is nothing in the neighborhood," remarked one contemporary observer to another, who retorted, "There never will be so long as you keep that madhouse there."[10] "No one outside the twenty-six governors of the New York Hospital," sarcastically noted a onetime state senator, "would dare to maintain that lunatics are desirable neighbors."[11] Others noted that "the governors say the lunatics don't injure or annoy anybody, because the region is desolate. That's the Gospel truth. That region will be desolate as long as the asylum is there. There will be no neighborhood, no development. People will not build houses in that locality so long as lunatics are stored in that madhouse." Speculators generally concluded that "the present location of Bloomingdale is a bar to public improvements, and is a black cloud hanging over a vast territory desirable for residential sites."[12]

The second major problem for real estate developers interested in the area was that the asylum and its land cut off their property from access to public transportation and therefore eliminated the usefulness of the land for tenement or apartment development. Before the development of the Broadway subway line, the upper reaches of Manhattan were connected to the developed portions of the city only by horse-drawn carriages that traveled up the Boulevard (later renamed Broadway) or by access to the Metropolitan Elevated Railroad line. This El traveled up Ninth Avenue to 110th Street and then curved over to Eighth Avenue, where it continued uptown to a stop at 116th Street. In the 1880s the El was the only public transportation available, and the 116th Street stop therefore had a special significance for speculators interested in developing residential housing. If the area was to be developed, access to this railroad stop had to be guaranteed.[13] As long as the asylum held onto its property and refused access to its grounds, residents on the West Side of the Boulevard were forced to circumvent the asylum in order to get to public transportation.

Throughout the mid-1880s numerous bills were introduced into the state assembly to support the building of public access routes through the asylum grounds at 116th and other streets from the Boulevard to Amsterdam Avenue.[14] But the governors defeated all efforts. "And now about those closed streets," declared one lobbyist seeking support for a bill to open 116th Street. "To whom do the streets belong – the people or the lunatics? . . . The opening of 116th Street alone would be a great boon." The reporter for the New York Herald noted that, in "deference to the public demand that 116th Street be cut through, this bill has been introduced for years, but the influence and social relations of the governors of the institution have always killed it."[15]

The interest of New York Hospital's governors in stifling commercial and residential development of the area emanated from a fear that such development would interfere with the asylum's functions as a refuge. They also feared that the real estate speculators, many of whom were Jewish, might cater to the growing immigrant population and turn Morningside Heights into a commercial and working-class residential district with the resulting complement of tenements, shacks, foundries, industries, and poverty. Such a change in the social and economic characteristics of the neighborhood was unacceptable to these merchants and bankers, who for years had been watching with dismay as the city they once controlled changed around them.

The governors of New York Hospital could not help but observe the signs of mass immigration, poverty, and suffering that seemed to engulf the city (see Table 11). Walking one block from the asylum, they could look out over Morningside Park and Harlem and observe the tenements going up in the distance near the Second and Third Avenue Els. There thousands of immigrants and their families were settling in New York's first "Little Italy" and in the German, Irish, and Jewish enclaves of East Harlem. By 1890 the character of East Harlem was already largely immigrant.

In some sections of the eastern portions of the Twelfth Ward, in which the asylum was located, over 85 percent of the population was composed of the foreign-born and their children. Twenty-three thousand of these people were jammed into 126 acres, an area only four times that controlled by the asylum on the west side. Just uptown from Little Italy was the Twelfth Ward's Sanitary District M, an area of 214 acres between East 110th Street and East 120th Street. This area was also dominated by tenements and light industry and held a population of nearly 40,000 in 1890. One hundred eighty-five persons lived on every acre of land in the eastern rim of the Twelfth Ward.[16] Not surprisingly, the area had a death rate well above the city's and suffered from extraordinary outbreaks of diphtheria, croup, diarrheal diseases, pneumonia, and other pulmonary and infectious illnesses.

The asylum, however, dominated the western portion of the Twelfth Ward. This area of 279 acres had only 17 persons living on each acre of land. Predictably, the health statistics for this region were substantially better than those of the eastern sections of the ward: The asylum's district had a death rate of only 16.7 per 1,000, whereas death rates in the eastern region were nearly 40 per 1,000.[17]

To the south, as well, immigrants and their children began to burst into new neighborhoods farther uptown. Whereas the upper West

Table 11. Selected demographic statistics for various sanitary districts in Wards 12 and 22 in Manhattan

	Death Rate	Population	Acres	No. of dwellings	Persons per acre	Persons per dwelling	% native-born	% foreign-born[a]	% black
Manhattan	31.01	1,515,301	25,818	81,828	58.69	18.52	17.8	80.5	1.7
Ward 12 (districts bordering asylum)									
S.D. A (W. 86–W. 94; Hudson–8th Ave.)	14.08	5,107	176	416	29.02	12.28	42.8	56.0	1.2
S.D. E (W. 102–W. 94; 8th Ave.–Hudson)	16.94	10,648	167	637	63.76	16.72	30.9	68.6	0.5
S.D. H (W. 110–W. 102; Hudson–8th Ave.)	14.74	6,669	168	365	43.03	18.27	35.4	63.4	1.2
S.D. L (W. & E. 110–W. & E. 120; 4th Ave.–7th Ave.)	16.64	7,471	166	530	45.01	14.10	31.3	68.0	0.7
S.D. N (W. 120–W. 130; 5th Ave.–Hudson)	20.19	25,744	385	—	70.73	—	38.9	59.0	2.1
S.D. K (W. 120–W. 110; 7th Ave.–Hudson; in-cluding asylum)	16.70	4,700	279	321	16.85	14.64	35.7	64.0	0.3

Ward 12 (East Harlem)

S.D. I (E. 110–E. 105; East River–5th Ave.)	40.65	23,358	126	1,012	185.38	23.08	15.0	84.8	0.2
S.D. M (E. 110–E. 120; East River–4th Ave.)	37.64	39,520	214	2,326	184.67	16.99	20.1	79.3	0.6

Ward 22 (West Side)

S.D. A (W. 40–W. 50; 10th Ave.–Hudson)	34.21	22,586	116	718	194.71	31.46	15.6	84.3	0.1
S.D. B (W. 40–W. 50; 8th Ave.–10th Ave.)	29.37	34,307	104	1,317	329.88	26.05	19.7	79.1	1.2
S.D. D (W. 50–W. 57; Hudson–10th Ave.)	36.86	10,007	75	443	133.00	22.50	15.0	83.9	1.1
S.D. G (W. 57–W. 64; 10th Ave.–Hudson)	40.80	10,237	80	234	127.96	43.75	10.3	82.2	7.5

Note: A dash indicates no data.

[a] Includes children of foreign-born and native-born children of parents either of whom were immigrants.

Source: Census Office, Department of the Interior, *Vital Statistics of New York City and Brooklyn, Covering a Period of Six Years Ending May 31, 1890* (Washington, D.C.: Government Printing Office, 1894).

Side was still a primarily middle- and upper-class area with a relatively large American-born population, the West Side below 64th Street was largely poor and Irish. More than 10,000 persons, over 82 percent of whom were immigrants, and their families were jammed into the 80-acre area between West Fifty-seventh and West Sixty-fourth streets, from Tenth Avenue to the Hudson River. An average of 44 people lived in each of the 234 tenements that dominated the district. The large slaughterhouses and breweries near the river further marred the area, the poverty of which was reflected in a death rate of over 40 per 1,000, nearly a third higher than that of the city as a whole.[18]

As immigrants moved uptown, control over land use appeared to be one of the last significant means of determining the future development of the city. Through the power inherent in land ownership and control, the established elites might preserve the traditional relationships between classes and religious groups – relationships that were quickly changing under the weight of immigration, industrialization, political bossism, and urbanization. By keeping the immigrant population from settling in certain areas of the city through land-use restrictions, the merchant and banking families in control of the boardrooms of charitable institutions might stop or at least stall the demise of the social order to which they were accustomed. In the absence of a city planning department or even professional urban planners, the boardroom of the hospital became a significant center for social and neighborhood planning and control.

The battle over Bloomingdale

> Will Bloomingdale Asylum Go? How long is that institution to retard the development of that beautiful section of the city . . . ? These and a lot of cognate queries are being asked by property owners . . . and particularly by gentlemen who comprise the Morningside Park Association. These gentlemen have taken off their coats, metaphorically speaking, and rolled up their sleeves and mean to fight Bloomingdale Insane Asylum for all it and they are worth.[19]

The battle between local real estate speculators and the governors of New York Hospital's Bloomingdale Asylum came to a head in the late 1880s. The asylum's governors had been promising to move from Morningside Heights for at least twenty-three years, since the end of the Civil War. As early as December 1866, the governors had "resolved that the present condition of the Asylum grounds, the probable occupation of adjoining land for building and other purposes, and the possible opening of streets through the Asylum grounds at no remote date" made it imperative that the governors seek land "for the Institution beyond the City limits."[20] But this early decision had not been acted upon. In fact, it appeared to many that the asylum would not move except under extraordinary political pressure. Beginning in the late 1880s, just such pressure was exerted by real estate speculators and their political allies. In late 1887, Democrats in the legislature began a serious and prolonged campaign to get the hospital to abandon its Morningside Heights land and leave Manhattan entirely. Initially the Democrats chose a traditional legislative attack and sought to enact laws allowing public access roads through the asylum grounds. They argued that such roads were necessary if the neighborhood was to be opened for development. On January 17, 1888, John Connelly, the assemblyman from the city's upper West Side, introduced an act to "lay out and improve One Hundred and Sixteenth Street from Tenth Avenue to the road and public drive known as the Broadway Boulevard." This meant that a public access street would be cut directly through the property of the Bloomingdale Asylum, leveling two small asylum buildings in the process. The cost of this road, the bill added, should be borne by "all parties and persons, lands and tenements, which they may deem to be benefitted."[21]

Despite solid support from Assemblyman Connelly, the mayor, and nearly all the major newspapers, this bill met extraordinary opposition from the powerful governors of the hospital, who lobbied among upstate Republicans. "The bill . . . is still in the Assembly Committee of Cities," reported the *Herald* on March 8. "It has slept there for five weeks under the powerful soporific administered by Commodore Elbridge T. Gerry and the Board of Governors of that wealthy and money-making institution for the opulent insane."[22]

The battle was prolonged and vicious because the stakes on each side were very high. The assemblyman from the area had a definite interest in aligning with the real estate developers, who promised to add housing and constituents to his largely underpopulated ward. As of 1888, after all, John Connelly "represented a lot of empty lots," as Elbridge Gerry, the wealthy lobbyist for the hospital, undiplomatically pointed out. According to Gerry, "the district around 116th Street and Morningside and Riverside Avenues was a howling wilderness and did not require any more streets." But Connelly and "the property owners" saw things differently. They "answered that the whole west side was booming except right there" in the neighborhood of the asylum.[23]

When it became apparent that the bill was tied up, all attempts at compromise and accommodation appeared hopeless, given the determination on both sides. Even mediation attempts made in early 1888 by New York City's Mayor Hewitt were fruitless. In early February, for instance, the mayor and one of the hospital's attorneys, Charles Strong of the Wall Street firm of Strong and Calwalader, met together to seek some compromise. The mayor argued that the bill to open the street was one that the hospital should accept, because the hospital's opposition would further solidify the power of its enemies. He pointed out that opposition might provoke the hospital's enemies to push for an even more extensive bill calling for the opening of 117th, 118th, and 119th streets as well. The opening of 117th Street, in particular, would demand the destruction of the asylum's main building. As Strong reported in a letter to Elbridge Gerry, the mayor "stated that by not opposing the bill [to open 116th Street], we would make a bargain with its advocates by which they would agree not to claim the opening of streets North of 116th Street which the hospital might desire to remain closed." If the hospital dropped its opposition, the mayor promised, he could almost guarantee that "the street would not be opened until it was absolutely necessary, and the hospital was perfectly ready to do so."[24] But Elbridge Gerry and the other governors saw no reason to compromise at the time and ignored the mayor's pleas.

Connelly and others seeking the removal of the asylum stepped up their attack. On February 9, only three days after Strong's meeting with the mayor, Connelly, Dwight Olmstead, and Francis M. Bixby, a former state senator, indicated that they would begin to investigate the asylum's status as a tax-exempt charitable institution. Acting with the support of the Morningside Park Association, the legislators claimed that not only was the asylum inhibiting the development of the West Side, but it was also bilking the city of thousands of dollars because of its tax-exempt status. "Will the Bloomingdale Asylum go?" asked one newspaper columnist. "How long is that institution to retard the development of that beautiful section of the city between Riverside and Morningside Parks? . . . Have the owners of adjacent property any right which the magnates of the Asylum are bound to respect?" The representatives of the Morningside Park Association, most particularly ex-Senator Bixby, who owned a fair amount of property in the area, joined with authors of the various street-construction bills to push for an investigation of the asylum's tax status. "Bloomingdale Asylum . . . gets the benefit of the taxes we pay," he noted, "but doesn't pay any taxes itself . . . We claim the institution is not a charity and is not conducted as such and that . . . the New York Hospital ought to pay taxes on its property."[25]

The legislators argued that the asylum served only the rich, who paid handsomely for their care; the poor, who should have been the recipients of charity services, were excluded. "Not in five years [has the asylum] taken a free patient," claimed Bixby. The asylum, he and others contended, "was simply a house for aristocratic lunatics."[26]

The popular press bolstered the attempts of the real estate people to portray the asylum in this way. In very short order, it depicted the asylum as nothing more than a money-making institution where services and expenditures for the "wealthy insane" were "the most lavish in the world." The press claimed that patients paid over $100 a week for their care and that poor persons, even asylum staff members, were turned away and sent to city institutions when they became mentally ill. The story developed that the occasional poor person who managed to get service from the asylum was housed in the basement, not in the luxurious private quarters. "I have long ago learned that in the law, in the administration of charities . . . there is one law for the rich and another for the poor," remarked one real estate owner.[27]

The governors of the hospital were depicted as little more than merciless profiteers who had "created a trust of $10,000,000 or $12,000,000 of valuable real estate." The papers pointed out that there was "nothing whatever to prevent them whenever they may see fit [from] winding up the affairs of the New York Hospital Society and dividing its vast estate."[28] Not only did the asylum's governors serve only the wealthy, said the press, but they were probably going to enjoy enormous profits at the expense of the sick. Given the propaganda, it is hardly surprising that Bixby even threatened to seek the arrest of the hospital's governors and president, Cornelius N. Bliss, who was also chairman of the Republican State Committee, for profiteering and maintaining a public nuisance. "I am in favor of immediately bringing suit for damages," said Bixby, "and arresting some of the governors. I own the lots on Morningside Hill . . . that are worth now $8,000 apiece. They would be worth $25,000 or $30,000 more at least if the asylum was removed." Concluded the reporter for the *New York World*, "Owing to the high social and business standing of the officers . . . a profound sensation would be created" by their arrest.[29]

The agitation in the popular press had a tremendous impact. From March 9 to May 5, 1888, the New York State Senate Committee on Taxation and Retrenchment carried out an investigation of the asylum's tax-exempt status. Under pressure from the Morningside Park Association, the committee spent days hearing testimony from a number of real estate speculators interested in the removal of the asylum. Members of the real estate firm of Lespinasse and Friedman and the brokerage house of Scott and Meyers testified that the asylum impeded access to the El and depressed land values and development in the area. As owners and developers of land in Harlem, then a primarily Jewish area, these developers saw the potential for growth.[30] Leopold Friedman of Lespinasse and Friedman publicly testified that he would gladly pay $6,000 apiece for the asylum lots, but the offer was turned down firmly.[31]

The charge against the asylum was simple. It was claimed "that the Bloomingdale Asylum, far from being a charitable institution is a private, money making concern that holds a large block of property . . . on which it should pay taxes."[32] The hospital seemed to be in trouble, and during the ensuing months Elbridge Gerry and other trustees stepped up the lobbying effort. Gerry, whose strong alliance with important Republican senators and representatives was well known, lobbied hard to gain a favorable report from the senate Committee on Taxation when it began its investigation in March of 1888.[33] But the "governors . . . were too secretive in their way of doing business," it was claimed, and the senate's investigatory committee descended upon the city.[34] As the agency granting tax exemption to the asylum, the senate, it was held, had the duty and the right to investigate the economic class of the asylum's patients and the means of financing the institution.

The attack on the tax status of the hospital was merely part of the larger battle to get the asylum off the Morningside land. The Morningside Park Association made this fact clear by incorporating earlier attempts to open up streets through the asylum into its petition to the senate pressing for the investigation. The association asked the senate to determine "whether or not any of the streets originally laid out through the asylum grounds at Bloomingdale, which are now closed to the public, should be opened," and "whether or not said lunatic asylum is detrimental to property in the neighborhood, or unsafe for persons residing or who might reside there, and whether the said asylum should be permitted to continue in that location."[35]

Those lobbying for the hospital argued differently. The governors claimed that the institution was neither a detriment to the community nor the reason that land values in the area appeared to be low. They also claimed that the asylum's tax-exempt status should be considered in the context of the hospital's charitable character: The tax exemption had been granted to the entire hospital, of which the asylum was only one branch. The governors maintained that the committee, when deciding on the tax question, should take into account the large amount of charitable work done free for indigent patients at the hospital's major branch on Fifteenth and Sixteenth streets.

In May the committee issued its report. The five senators on the committee split in their recommendations. The majority, three upstate senators, agreed with the hospital, saying that the work of the asylum could not be divorced from the charitable work of the hospital itself. Furthermore, the majority contended that the asylum itself was not detrimental to the neighborhood, and that its land should not have streets cut through it, because so few persons lived in the area. The minority of downstate senators vehemently disagreed with these conclusions and called for the building of streets through the land, removal of the asylum from the city, and the immediate taxation of its Morningside lots.[36] The report of the committee appeared to be a major victory for the hospital.

The victory celebration was short-lived, however. On the same day the Committee on Taxation reached its conclusions, another senate committee, the Committee on Cities, published a favorable report on the opening of various streets. Although this bill did not itemize the streets to be opened, the hospital governors realized that this was yet another attack by the real estate speculators on the asylum. "I see by last evening's paper that Senator Langbine's [sic] bill for opening streets in the City of New York was reported favorably," wrote Charles Strong, the hospital's lawyer, to Elbridge Gerry. "Are you aware what this bill is? . . . As he [Langbein] is the author of the [Committee on Taxation's] minority report in the case of the Asylum, it occurs to me that it might be possible that he is endeavoring to reach the opening of 116th Street by another method than the bill which you killed."[37]

Strong was correct. Senator Langbein and others interested in opening the Morningside land to development were indeed endeavoring to reach their goals by other means. Furthermore, during the battle over the taxation report, the governors had called in a great number of political debts. Now their political clout was eroded. After the Committee on Taxation's report, the hospital faced more, not less, pressure to move.

By the beginning of 1889 it was apparent that the Bloomingdale Asylum would finally have to leave the city or be closed. The combined forces of the Morningside Park Association, downstate assemblymen and senators, the mayor, the Democratic Party machine, and most of the city's newspapers were too much even for the prestigious board of governors. In late 1888 it became obvious that the lobbying efforts of Elbridge Gerry were going to be inadequate, and the hospital turned for help to Cornelius Bliss, a member of the board of governors and the president of the Republican State Committee. By doing so, they played their last card and made the battle over the street opening a strictly partisan one.[38] But this move only brought further criticism. As one real estate broker said, the "governors . . . are becoming very unpopular on the West Side – especially since the Republic State Committee has taken a hand in [their] affairs." In the press as well, Gerry and other governors were denounced as "aristocratic lobbyists" and "contemptible rattlesnakes" for using pure political muscle to protect the asylum's location.[39]

Republicans began to weaken in their support of the hospital. State senators could not continue to ignore its tremendous unpopularity in New York City. When the governors pressed a friendly assemblyman named Hornsby to introduce an early version of a tax-exemption bill, they were met with a demure apology: "I do not see how I can introduce it and should like to be relieved. I got into trouble last year by introducing an exemption bill for Mr. Charles E. Strong and was attacked by the newspapers." He protested that he did "not mind criticism but I think in this case it would be just. The feeling against the exemption is strong and growing and I rather share in it . . . When I spoke to you, I did not appreciate the full effect of the bill and I must reluctantly ask you to give it to some one else."[40]

The governors had little choice but to prepare to move the asylum from Manhattan to hospital property in the town of White Plains in Westchester, New York. While continuing to oppose the attacks on the Bloomingdale Asylum, the lobbyist for the hospital began a concerted effort in the senate and assembly to gain tax-exempt status for the Westchester land. No sooner had the legislators returned from their Christmas break early in 1889 than they were hit with the competing bills of hospital and real estate spokesmen. In the senate one bill called for the opening of all streets between 116th and 120th, and another demanded the "assessment and taxation of certain real estate [in the Morningside Park area] owned by the Society of New York Hospital."[41] In the assembly, an act to open 116th Street was introduced by Assemblyman Connelly, and a Westchester senator introduced another bill to exempt the properties of New York Hospital from taxation. In the meantime, the hospital's real estate and law committees prepared for the inevitable move by selling portions of its uptown land at auction.[42]

The bill to seek tax exemption for the White Plains land was seen as crucial for the orderly transfer of the asylum from Manhattan. In fact, it was so important that Gerry and Bliss lobbied intensively for the measure, and Strong, the hospital's attorney, drafted and circulated two petitions calling for the legislature to pass the tax-exemption bills when they came up. As early as December 1888, Strong informed Gerry of the petitions, ostensibly from Westchester residents, and sent him copies. Some "of the influential people at White Plains wish to assist us in this matter [and] I concluded to amend the one [petition] which I prepared so it would ask for the exemption without assigning any reasons," Strong reported.[43] By February, given the strong opposition to the hospital, both Gerry and Bliss were called upon to lobby hard in Albany. Wrote Charles Nichols, the asylum's superintendent, "I do not know how strong Commodore Gerry's confidence is, nor very much of the grounds of his confidence whatever it be, that the tax-exemption bill will become a law . . . but [as] there be much doubt of its prompt passage I think the two gentlemen" – Bliss and Gerry – should "combine [in] a tower of strength" to force its passage.[44]

Meanwhile, the bill to open 116th Street passed the assembly on March 29, 1889. It was amended in the Senate and passed in the middle of May, over the frustrated objections of Gerry and Republican senators who, at the time of its passage, hardly realized that the Democrats had engineered it through. An upset Gerry reported to the president of the society the day after the bill's passage:

> Upon the assurance of Mr. Bliss, that Connelly's bill would not be reported out of the Cities Committee, I paid no attention to the matter while up at Albany. But on Wednesday night, the day before adjournment, [the] Chairman of the Committee suddenly reported in a low voice three bills, two of which were immediately passed and the title to the third was read so indistinctly by the clerk that I did not catch it." [On] looking up [I] saw Mr. Connelly standing near Mr. Ives, and immediately suspected mischief. I jumped forward and attracted the attention of Senator Vedder [a supporter of the Hospital], who went forward to the clerk and found that it was the . . . bill, amended in Committee to take effect in 1894. I went at once to the Assembly and endeavored to stop the bill there against concurrence, but in the disorder in which that body was, it was simply impossible . . . I lodged a protest with [Governor Hill's] Secretary on the subject.[45]

There seemed little hope, however, that the governor would veto this bill, which had now passed both houses.

The passage of the street bill made the hospital tax-exemption bill of even greater concern for the trustees. This bill to exempt the Westchester site from taxation had already passed the legislature at this point, and was sitting on the governor's desk awaiting his signature. He had until the middle of June to sign both the exemption bill and the street-opening bill. The hospital and Governor Hill, of course, saw the two bills, which had passed both houses of the legislature on the same day, as part of a larger political compromise between the asylum and the pro-real estate interests. The two bills, when taken together, gave the asylum until 1894 to vacate its uptown Manhattan site and move to tax-exempt land in Westchester County. The hospital would have four years to erect the Westchester Asylum and leave Manhattan.[46]

The power of the hospital's board of governors had rested in its close alliance with the Republican Party, and the enormous prestige and power of some of its members. Bliss, a banker and important member of the board of governors, was head of the Republican State Committee during the period when the battle took place and head of the Republican National Committee a few years later. Both positions indicate his importance in Republican politics. Gerry, a member of the board of governors and the hospital's principal lobbyist in Albany, was from an established Republican family. His grandfather had signed the Declaration of Independence and was vice-president under James Madison. His father, Elbridge Gerry II, had been a member of the House of Representatives in Maine and, later, a Republican senator from Massachusetts. Gerry's father had been instrumental in reapportioning party power in Massachusetts to the Republicans by altering the voting district: The term "gerrymander" was a lingering reminder to all Republicans of his importance in Republican politics.[47]

But the hospital's quest to control the use of the land on the West Side was doomed as long as its only alternative to urban development was maintaining the status quo. The power of the real estate forces was too strong and the value of the land too great for the policy of resistance to succeed. By 1889 it was clear that the asylum would have to move, and the governors, forced to abandon direct ownership, sought new methods for controlling the social character of the neighborhood they were leaving.

Land use and social control on Morningside Heights

By the middle of March 1889, the hospital was auctioning off miscellaneous lots of land in the uptown area. The parcels on 112th, 113th, and 114th streets were sold quickly, but the hospital governors were careful to retain the holdings between 114th and 120th streets, where the asylum stood. Although the previous battle had apparently been over the hospital's right to maintain the asylum there, it quickly became clear that, for the governors, there was another very significant issue: How could they ensure that, in selling this land, they did not let power pass from the elites they represented to the real estate interests and the immigrant classes that were increasingly trying to assume control?

A legal covenant signed by the hospital's representatives and buyers when the lots on 112th, 113th, and 114th streets were sold clearly indicates the extent to which the governors wished to control the future development of the area. The covenant delineated what could and could not be done to the property by the new owners. It stated that the Society of New York Hospital would sell the land subject to restrictions on the kinds of buildings to be erected and the purposes for which they could be used. The hospital would not permit, for a "period of twenty years from the date of" the sale, any

> railroad depot or car house, smith shop, carpenter shop, livery stable, foundry or manufactory of any kind, bone boiling establishment, nor any establishment for the tanning, dressing, or preparing of skins, hides, or leather, nor any brewery or distillery nor establishment for refining or storing oil or petroleum, nor any other noxious, dangerous or offensive trade, occupation or business, nor any houses commonly known as tenement houses.[48]

By these restrictions, the hospital sought to ensure that the area developed as a noncommercial, residential neighborhood for people who would travel away from it to work.

The covenants were designed to ensure the construction of middle-class housing. Apartment buildings would be allowed as long as they consisted "of a suite of rooms upon single floors . . . adapted and intended each as the residence of a single family." Because it was possible that tenement apartments designed for working-class populations might be built within the criteria set down for apartments, the governors placed further stipulations on apartment construction: Apartment buildings would be allowed only on the avenues (Broadway and Columbus), and all housing in between would be reserved for those of substantially greater personal wealth. All housing "100 feet Westerly from the Westerly line of 10th Avenue and . . . 100 feet Easterly from the Easterly line of the Boulevard," the covenant decreed, "shall only be first class private dwelling houses of brick, or stone, with roofs of slate, tin or other metal or any fire proof material, and not less than 4 stories in height, and designed for the occupancy of a single family each." The hospital thereby guaranteed that, for the following twenty years, only expensive brownstone and whitestone townhouses for individual families could be built on the land it was selling. No industry and no working-class housing would be allowed.[49]

Even these covenants, however, could not prevent the construction of commercial establishments on adjacent pieces of land never owned by the hospital or on the former hospital land after the twenty-year term of the covenant had expired. Unless a powerful and stable tenant could be found to establish the desired upper-middle-class character of the neighborhood, there was still a possibility that immigrant groups could take over. The Cathedral of St. John the Divine was already planned for the site on Tenth Avenue (recently renamed Amsterdam Avenue), and Grant's Tomb was planned for construction in Riverside Park. If another major institution of established reputation could be found for the asylum's major tract of land, then the character of the area as an elite Protestant enclave in an increasingly Catholic and Jewish city might be permanently established.

In late 1891, representatives of Columbia College approached the hospital's governors. The college, then crammed into a small area on Madison Avenue at Fiftieth Street, was in need of a larger area, farther away from the traffic noise and railroad terminals. In November 1891, Seth Low, then president of Columbia, wrote a confidential letter to Herman H. Cammann, chairman of the hospital's Real Estate Committee and a major real estate broker. In the letter Low described the needs of his institution and remarked that he and William Schermerhorn had been appointed to "enquire whether the New York Hospital would give to Columbia College an option on the property now occupied by the Bloomingdale Asylum, bounded east and west by 10th Avenue and the Boulevard and lying between 116th and 120th Streets." Low asked for the option to "fix as distant a date as possible at which Columbia would be expected to take possession in case of a purchase."[50]

When Low emphasized that he approached the governors "frankly, believing that in this spirit alone is it possible for anything to be done between us," he was acknowledging a kind of fellowship among powerful Protestant-controlled interests. He suggested that the financially strained college and the politically defeated hospital could assist each other. "We understand that at least a very large sum of money is involved," Low wrote, "and it remains to be determined, after the details have been agreed upon between us, whether Columbia can justly use so large a sum for this purpose. This is a question hard to answer in the abstract and comparatively easy to answer when it is definite. I hope that the Board of Governors," he concluded, " in considering my question and in naming a price, will not forget the public character of Columbia College, and its usefulness to the City of New York and the whole country."[51]

The board of governors of the hospital jumped at the college's discreet inquiry. One month after Low's letter, on December 2, they offered the land between 116th and 120th streets to Columbia for $2 million. In January 1892 Columbia published a "Statement of the Committee on Site" calling for removal of the college from the midtown site and its relocation on the Bloomingdale land. In order to garner financial support for the move from the alumni, the statement emphasized that the land between Morningside and Riverside parks was "among the most beautiful which the City affords." Furthermore, the "Cathedral of St. John the Divine and the Grant Monument are to be erected upon the same plateau and within a few blocks of the proposed site, [and] if Columbia should be enabled to develop the property to its full possibilities, the locality would become a part of the City which every stranger would visit and of which every citizen would be proud."[52] The sale of this land to Columbia would guarantee the land's domination by prestigious public and private institutions of which the upper classes of the city could be proud. With the sale, the board of governors felt that they fulfilled their social obligation to maintain control over the city by participating in the governance of these institutions. Columbia's $2 million also aided the hospital, of course, but perhaps most important, this arrangement kept the real estate speculators who had opposed the governors from gaining access to this valuable portion of the city. The deal between Columbia and the New York Hospital was all but finalized in a period of two months.

Seth Low's social and class connections had certainly facilitated the transfer of the land to Columbia College. Low had graduated from Columbia and was a descendant of a wealthy merchant family. His long ties to the Republican Party dated back to his election as a Republican mayor of Brooklyn in 1881. In the 1880s Low had emerged as a major advocate of "efficiency" in local government. He maintained that "it was almost impossible for the average resident to participate constructively in the affairs of the city," and argued that only educated and nonpartisan officials should have the responsibility for important political decisions.[53] Unlike the older "gentry," who held the immigrants or their representatives responsible for the inefficiency and corruption of the city government, Low maintained that the problems of governance were structural in nature and resided in the methods of governmental administration and the qualifications of those in power. He felt that control over the city should depend not upon who controlled the political machine but upon who controlled the departments of city government. Rather than supporting popular elections for civil service positions, Low advocated that greater authority be given to the mayor's office to appoint and remove department heads at his discretion. For

Low, control of the city should not be a matter of back-ward politics or aristocratic inheritance; it should be based upon experience and education, qualities that were then the province of the older elites.[54]

The significance of Low's views could not have escaped the hospital's board of governors. Low, after all, had been mayor of Brooklyn and was now head of Columbia College. In a few years he would leave Columbia to become a reform mayor of New York City itself. That the hospital governors decided in such a short time to sell to Columbia signified a trust in the institution and its leader that went beyond monetary interests alone. For this older group of merchants and gentry, Columbia represented the last hope for the long-term hegemony of the elite.

In many ways the struggle for control of the New York Hospital land reflected the political and ideological debates then being waged between upper- and working-class groups. The older charity hospital had by this time lost a fair amount of social legitimacy, as politicians, newspapers, and immigrant groups attacked it for the aristocratic pretensions of its governing group. Its hierarchical organization and paternalistic governance merely added to its image as an antidemocratic, anti–working-class institution.

Columbia College, on the other hand, had greater social legitimacy. As an educational institution, it was less susceptible to charges that it was aristocratic and antidemocratic in organization and governance. Its educational objectives, indeed, were consistent with popular democratic images of self-improvement and advancement by merit. Although most nineteenth-century New Yorkers perceived Columbia as the province of wealthy elites, education in and of itself was not seen as inherently antidemocratic.

The governors' desire to maintain Morningside Heights as an upper-middle-class residential area went beyond their restrictions on construction and controls over land sales. Even after they had divested themselves of major portions of their real estate in the area, they continued their attempts to control the development of that area. All forms of attack by the commercializing forces from lower Manhattan were met with strong and concerted opposition. In 1897, for instance, a trolley company sought to build a trolley service on Amsterdam Avenue, then adjacent to the hospital's remaining acreage between 114th and 116th streets and to land now occupied by Columbia, St. John the Divine, and other educational and religious institutions. It was quickly observed that trolleys would disrupt the residential, religious, and collegiate atmosphere of this neighborhood. The Board of Governors of New York Hospital combined with the presidents and officials of Columbia, Teachers College, Barnard College, the Cathedral of St. John the Divine, Riverside Church, and a number of other local institutions to make a protest, and joined the "Amsterdam Avenue Anti-Grab Committee," then known as the "People's Committee," to fight the trolleys. This committee attempted "to prevent the running of four lines of trolley cars on Amsterdam Avenue, which would certainly ruin the thoroughfare for residential purposes." The hospital sent the princely sum of $500 to support the legal battle.[55]

These attempts to control the use of land in the Morningside Heights area must be understood within the context of the shifting political and social scene in late-nineteenth-century New York. At this time, an ongoing political battle for control over the life of the city was in progress among an older merchant class, the Tammany Hall ward bosses, and a rising group of upper-class reformers. In general, old-line merchant families, primarily Republicans, sought to maintain their traditional social and political position in the face of the tremendous power of the Tammany Hall Democrats and their immigrant constituents. As new immigrants and their Tammany leaders began to dominate local politics, it became apparent that control of the important aspects of the city's life was slipping from their grasp. Within this context, control over land use became especially important.

The city appeared to be changing in ways inconceivable to members of the merchant class, many of whom had only to think back to their childhood to remember a smaller, more homogeneous city that their families dominated socially, politically, and economically. The changes overtaking New York were clearly threatening to this older group of merchants and gentry. The political life of the city was now dominated by Irish Catholic politicians and other foreign-born "bosses." Furthermore, the new industrialists and robber barons, with their increasing wealth, threatened the economic supremacy of the older merchants.

The demographic and physical makeup of the city was perhaps the most obvious indication of the changing nature of urban life. Not only had factories and industries arisen in Brooklyn, the East River area, and the lower West Side, but tenements and other forms of housing for the millions of arriving immigrants spread throughout the city. The lower East Side had long been a neighborhood of immigrants. But by the 1880s the upper East Side, Harlem, and the upper West Side were dotted with tenements housing Jewish, Italian, Irish, and other immigrants.

With the massive Eastern European and Irish immigration, and the development of strong ethnic communities in the 1870s and 1880s, political power shifted substantially within local government. Those who had previously controlled the mayor's office and other governmental posts increasingly found ward bosses and a powerful immigrant-dominated Democratic Party assuming substantial control over many elected positions. From a position of political power, these newly elected officials were able to disperse the spoils of patronage to their constituents, thus strengthening the hand of the Tammany Hall leaders who controlled the party. By the 1880s the control of New York's political life had passed from old-line patricians to newer party professionals, who were largely Irish or members of some other ethnic group.[56]

The older gentry who dominated the boards of many large charitable hospitals looked upon these changes with a jaundiced eye. They feared the growing power of the ward bosses and were convinced that working-class groups were incapable of governing effectively. Often insensitive to the growing needs of the arriving immigrants for housing and other social services, these older elites sought ways to undermine the power base of the developing immigrant communities and to maintain control of the growing city. Two widely recognized aspects of the attack by industrial elites were the political reform efforts and a growing emphasis on efficiency in government and public education.[57]

But for older merchants and bankers on the boards of charitable institutions, the attempt at social control extended to other areas of everyday life as well. It has been widely recognized that the nineteenth-century hospital emphasized religious education and moral teachings for the hospital's working-class patients. Hospital trustees' visiting committees, nurses, and nuns often used the institution as a center for undermining the beliefs and culture of patients housed therein. Through moral training and requirements that turned them into orderlies and laundry and dietary room workers during long hospital stays, patients were made to see themselves as the recipients of paternal attention. But socializing and reforming hospital patients was only one means by which the hospital exercised social control. As we have seen in the case of New York Hospital, hospital trustees and administrators sought to control the economic structure and the social-class characteristics of an entire section of the city. The governors of New York Hospital acted partly out of financial need, partly out of fear of the changes occurring within the city, and partly out of a belief in the obligation of their class to prevent what they perceived as the destruction of a city by forces of urbanization, immigration, and industrialization.

8 Looking backward

By the end of the Progressive era, Manhattan and Brooklyn had gone through a radical transformation. Clearly, Brooklyn was no longer the "City of Churches" nor the "City of Homes." Its nineteenth-century rural, bucolic flavor was gone. Manhattan had become the center of finance and industry for the entire country. New York was a highly industrial, crowded city with a large portion of its population composed of immigrants and their children.

Manhattan, the home for millions of immigrants, thousands of banks and commercial enterprises, and a score of millionaires, became the undisputed economic capital of an increasingly powerful country. Brooklyn, once known for Henry Ward Beecher and his Plymouth Church, became known for its massive bridges and factories. Even the local baseball team had to change its name to conform to the new reality. The Brooklyn Robins, named for the team's original owner, became the Brooklyn Dodgers by the 1920s, as trolley dodging became a widespread popular sport and as robins were replaced by pigeons in the downtown area. Soon the Dodgers would be nicknamed the Brooklyn "Bums," in a further reflection of the growing city's urban, working-class character.

It is paradoxical, perhaps, that just as New York was emerging as a working-class city, its charity and other health institutions began to turn away form the poor and to remodel their services around the needs of wealthier clients. The spatial reorganization of the city, prompted by the introduction of the trolley, the subway, and the telephone and the resultant commercialization of the downtown area, forced doctors to move their offices far away from poorer neighborhoods. The financial crisis of the various hospitals caused trustees in these institutions to deny service to the poorest and most needy and to shunt the traditional "charity" cases off to the public institutions. Governmental reorganization destroyed the financial structure of those small hospitals close to the working class, and a combination of city and state actions undermined the viability of the local dispensaries.

These changes had dire long-term consequences for the delivery of health services to the city's poor and working-class groups. First, voluntary hospital care was reorganized around the needs of wealthier

November, 1917
Vol. IV, No. 4

HOSPITAL MANAGEMENT

608 S. Dearborn Street, Chicago

Published in the Interest of Executives in Every Department of Hospital Work
Entered as second class matter May 14, 1917, at the post office at Chicago, Ill., under the act of March 3, 1879.

Hospital Service Must Balance Needs of Patient

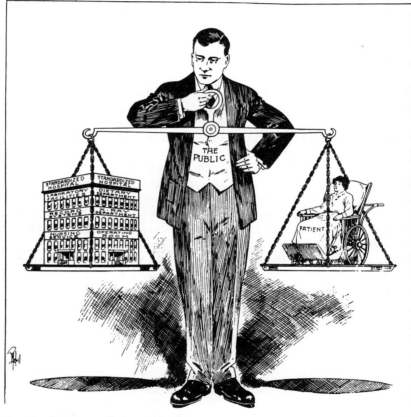

Standardization and efficiency often seemed to become goals unto themselves. Here *Hospital Management* reminds its readers that, to satisfy the public, the hospital will have to meet the needs of the patient as well. Many of the illustrations periodically published in the journal reminded the reader that the goals of business and medical efficiency should not overwhelm the hospital's social functions as a humanitarian enterprise.

clients who demanded private rooms. Internally, institutions became differentiated according to social class, as poorer patients went to public institutions, were kept in "free" wards, or were forced to pay for "better-quality" care in paying wards. Slightly wealthier clients were given private wards and rooms in which they had the option of receiving a variety of extra services, including better food, private-duty nursing and private physician care. Hospitals became dependent upon the services of private physicians, who provided them with needed private and paying patients.

All of these social changes were taking place within the context of a rapidly changing medical and scientific environment. Doctors, administrators, trustees, and patients were often profoundly optimistic about the possibilities of changing medical practice. Within this context, the changes in health care were seen as progressive and necessary by those closest to the centers of power. Hospitals were refurbished; highly differentiated specialty services were added; and scientific practitioners began to set the goals and define the direction of and new standards for the health system. Within this atmosphere, small, low-technology, understaffed, freestanding ambulatory-care centers were seen as obsolete. Local hospitals and small institutions were judged unnecessary. Home- or office-based doctors' practices were regarded as an inefficient luxury that needed to be protected while members of the profession began a long-term migration to relocate their practices in the hospitals. From the perspective of Progressive era America, these changes in the health system were necessary and good. Also, because change in health care was extremely uneven, the broader implications of the seemingly idiosyncratic redirection of individual institutions were easy for most people to ignore.

But from our present perspective, the redirection was perhaps tragic. The chance to develop a viable set of freestanding ambulatory-care centers in poorer neighborhoods disappeared. The opportunity to make social services an intrinsic and important part of health-care delivery vanished. The opportunity to develop health-care services responsive to local community interests was lost. Indeed, the very class distinctions that characterized relationships in the outside society were brought into the hospital and came to characterize distinctions in services.

The health system, perhaps more than other areas of social service, reflects the dominant values and interests of a society. As we saw at the beginning of this book, the nineteenth-century hospital was built to resemble a home, or a church. By the 1920s, a new hospital looked

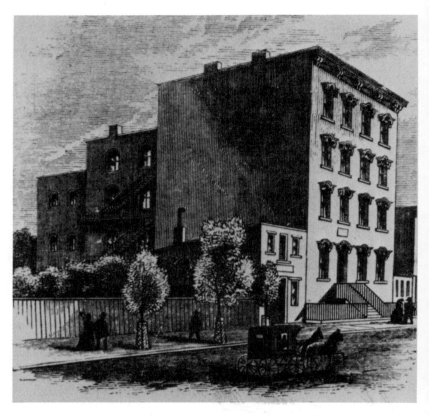

The first Mount Sinai Hospital: the Jews' Hospital on West Twenty-eighth Street.

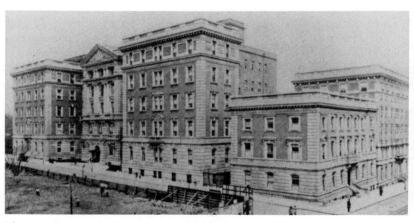

The new Mount Sinai Hospital on Fifth Avenue, 1904.

more like a factory, a hotel, or an apartment building. The structures of both periods reflect their historical moment, their inspiration, and the interests that built them. In November 1916 the *Modern Hospital*, "A Monthly Journal Devoted to the Building, Equipment, and Administration of Hospitals . . . ," devoted its lead story to the reconstruction of Brooklyn Hospital. Entitled "Brooklyn's Oldest Hospital Built Anew," the article detailed the floor-by-floor reorganization of the facility. A detailed plan of every story of every wing attested to the efficiency of the new institution. The first page of the article displayed an engraving of the entire hospital complex, showing in the background the symbols of the new city: a factory pouring out smoke and the bridge leading to Manhattan. In the foreground stood the hospital, composed of two dominant wings with a smaller building in between. Across the roof of one wing was the word "PUBLIC"; across the roof of the other was the word "PRIVATE." Between these stood the administration building, keeping two worlds of medicine far apart.[1]

Notes on sources

The history of New York's and Brooklyn's health systems demanded research in a number of different kinds of source materials. I consulted various medical and public health archives, along with more traditional sources for social historians. For those specifically interested in institutional and professional history, the most useful materials for Brooklyn are available at the Downstate Medical College Library. Among its holdings are the daybooks of some important Brooklyn physicians, including Alexander Skene, the author of a widely used nineteenth-century text on gynecology and obstetrics, and various annual reports from Brooklyn's hospitals, charity associations, and dispensaries. The varied correspondence of Dr. Joseph Raymond, secretary of the Long Island College Hospital during the 1890s and early twentieth century, is available there, and the Downstate Library also holds many of the materials formerly kept at the Kings County Medical Society, including copies of directories, reports, and newsletters sent to its membership. Unfortunately, much of this collection is in extremely poor condition because of lack of funds and available space. Unless a serious restoration process is initiated, it may soon be lost to scholars.

Brooklyn has no central source for its medical and public health history. Much of the work required for this book was done at the institutions that have lasted until the present. The Jewish Hospital of Brooklyn, presently threatened with closure, has nearly all of its patient medical records, dating from the time of its opening, on microfilm. Demographic profiles of its patients can be developed from this source. The Brooklyn Hospital has an archive that includes its board of trustees minutes, various correspondence, annual reports, and other items of historical and antiquarian interest. Under the direction of Dr. Edwin Maynard, Jr., the archive should prove to be a useful source. The Methodist Hospital of Brooklyn still has its executive and board of trustees minutes, although there is not yet any attempt to develop an archive for the use of historians. Other Brooklyn institutions have a variety of materials in varying states of decay. These collections may be lost unless a serious effort is made to protect them.

The story in Manhattan is considerably brighter. The New York Academy of Medicine is, of course, the single best source for materials on particular physicians and hospitals and for other printed materials of interest to historians. The Archives of the New York Hospital–Cornell Medical Center under the direction of Adele A. Lerner and Lisa Hottin, assistant archivist, have a wealth of material on the hospital, including its board minutes, medical committee reports, and a host of other documents. In addition, the archives have items on a number of other institutions, some of which have been incorporated into the New York Hospital. The materials are extremely well preserved and accessible, and the work environment is excellent. Specific hospitals and medical schools, such as Columbia College of Physicians and Surgeons, have a variety of printed and manuscript documents, but by and large, they are not well preserved. The United Hospital Fund Library has some useful historical resources, including a good picture collection of various New York hospitals.

Public health materials can be gathered through the Haven Emerson Library at the Department of Health of the City of New York. The Municipal Archives and the Municipal Library both contain useful items, especially on the Department of Public Charities and its relations to the various hospitals and dispensaries in New York. Special reports and other useful resources on political developments are available as well. Some of these documents are also available through the New York Public Library at Forty-second Street and Columbia University's various collections. There are additional copies of the reports of the Department of Public Charities and the comptroller's reports at Harvard University's Widener Library.

Notes

Abbreviations used in the notes

BCD   Brooklyn City Dispensary
BMJ   *Brooklyn Medical Journal*
BDE   *Brooklyn Daily Eagle*
DSML   Downstate Medical College Library
JAMA   *Journal of the American Medical Association*
LICH   Long Island College Hospital
LIMJ   *Long Island Medical Journal*
NYH   New York Hospital
NYT   *New York Times*
NYTrib   *New York Tribune*

Introduction

1 From the *Jewish Forward*, June 6, 1909, translated in Irving Howe and Kenneth Libo (eds.), *How We Lived: A Documentary History of Immigrant Jews in America, 1880–1930* (New York: New American Library, 1979), p. 75.
2 See Howe and Libo, *How We Lived,* in which the editors correctly point out the importance of this hospital for building a "sense of community." The special origins of this institution made it a significantly less oppressive environment for its patients than were most other institutions of the period.
3 Charles Rosenberg, "Inward Vision and Outward Glance: The Shaping of the American Hospital, 1880–1914," *Bulletin of the History of Medicine,* 53 (Fall 1979), 346–391, provides a good overview of social relationships in the nineteenth-century hospital.
4 There are still important traditions that distinguish institutions sponsored by Catholic, Jewish, or Protestant groups, but these differences are much less pronounced than in the past. Many of today's significant differences relate less to the sponsors' social characteristics than to the size, educational programs, and specialty of the institution.
5 E. H. Lewinski-Corwin, *The Hospital Situation in Greater New York* (New York: Putnam, 1924), pp. 21–25, 41.
6 Ibid., pp. 37–39; for more current estimates, see Department of Health, Education, and Welfare, *Health – United States, 1978* (Washington, D.C.: Government Printing Office, 1978).
7 Lewinski-Corwin, *The Hospital Situation,* pp. 45–47.

8   Ibid., pp. 43–45; Lewinski-Corwin points out (pp. 43–44) that "the practice
    of designating an ordinary ward for semi-private patients is at times
    merely a means on the part of the hospital of obtaining additional income,
    without at the same time offering to the patients better services or more
    privacy than in the public wards."
9   Henry E. Sigerist, "An Outline of the Development of the Hospital,"
    Bulletin of the Institute of the History of Medicine, 4 (July 1936), 573–581. Sigerist
    ties the development of the modern hospital to the evolution of improved
    medical practice. See also, George Rosen, "The Hospital: Historical Soci-
    ology of a Community Institution," in George Rosen, *From Medical Police to
    Social Medicine* (New York: Science History, 1974), pp. 274–303. More
    recent work by Morris J. Vogel, *The Invention of the Modern Hospital: Boston,
    1870–1930* (Chicago: University of Chicago Press, 1980), has been a wel-
    come addition to the literature. Also see Charles Rosenberg, "And Heal
    the Sick: The Hospital and Patient in Nineteenth Century America,"
    Journal of Social History, 10 (June 1977), 428–447; and Paul Starr, *The Trans-
    formation of American Medicine* (New York: Basic, 1982). Another work that
    will prove extremely valuable is Susan Reverby, " 'Apprenticeship to
    Duty': The Rationalization of American Nursing, 1860–1940" (unpub-
    lished Ph.D. dissertation, Boston University, 1982). This work looks at the
    effect of nursing on hospital organization and the conflicts within the
    profession.
10 A good summary of the history of the medical profession and practice is
    John Duffy, *The Healers: The Rise of the American Medical Establishment* (New
    York: McGraw-Hill, 1976); see also Martin S. Pernick, *A Calculus of Suffer-
    ing: Pain and Anesthesia in Nineteenth Century Medicine* (New York: Columbia
    University Press, forthcoming).
11 See Duffy, *The Healers*, pp. 256–257.
12 Charles E. Rosenberg, *The Cholera Years: The United States in 1832, 1848 and
    1866* (Chicago: University of Chicago Press, 1962).
13 The vibrant public health movement grew in part out of the relationship
    between piety and health that was perceived in the nineteenth century.
    See, for example, Charles Rosenberg, "Piety and Social Action: Some
    Origins of the American Public Health Movement," in Rosenberg, *No
    Other Gods: On Science and American Thought* (Baltimore: Johns Hopkins Uni-
    versity Press, 1976), pp. 109–122.
14 There is an extensive literature on medical education reform. See, for
    example, Gerald E. Markowitz and David K. Rosner, "Doctors in Crisis:
    Medical Education and Medical Reform during the Progressive Era, 1895–
    1915," in Susan Reverby and David Rosner (eds.), *Health Care in America:
    Essays in Social History* (Philadelphia: Temple University Press, 1979), pp.
    185–205; Morris J. Vogel and Charles E. Rosenberg (eds.), *The Therapeutic
    Revolution: Essays in the Social History of American Medicine* (Philadelphia: Uni-
    versity of Pennsylvania Press, 1979); and Ronald Numbers (ed.), *The Edu-
    cation of the American Physician* (Berkeley and Los Angeles: University of
    California Press, 1980). There is currently a controversy over a more

recent book by E. Richard Brown, *Rockefeller Medicine Men: Medicine and Capitalism in America* (Berkeley and Los Angeles: University of California Press, 1979).

15 H. Jack Geiger, at a recent colloquium in honor of Martin Cherkasky from Montefiore Hospital ("Social Medicine: The Continuing Agenda," Rockefeller University, New York, May 28, 1981), likened the hospital to a satellite of the community.

16 See the Methodist Hospital *Annual Reports* for the 1890s, particularly for the year 1900, p. 17, in which the surgeons complain about the inadequacy of the surgical environment.

17 "Hospital Needs and Finances," *Charities*, 15 (Nov. 11, 1905), 212–218. See particularly the "Report of the Sub-Committee on Economy," pp. 213–214.

18 See Gert Brieger, "Surgery," in Numbers, *Education of the American Physician*, pp. 188–190.

19 John Thompson quoted this physician at Montefiore Hospital at "Social Medicine: The Continuing Agenda," Rockefeller University, May 28, 1981.

1. Health care and community change

1 There is an extensive literature on nineteenth-century communities and the process of change and suburbanization. See, for example, Robert Wiebe, *The Search for Order, 1877–1920* (New York: Hill & Wang, 1967); and Hutchins Hapgood, *The Spirit of the Ghetto*, ed. Moses Rischin (Cambridge, Mass.: Belknap Press/Harvard University Press, 1967).

2 Frederick M. Dearborn, *The Metropolitan Hospital: A Chronical of Sixty-Two Years* (New York: Private printing, 1937), p. 37.

3 Ibid., p. 38.

4 Ibid.

5 Ibid., p. 31.

6 Ibid., p. 47.

7 John Duffy, *The Healers: The Rise of the Medical Establishment* (New York: McGraw-Hill, 1976), pp. 228–236.

8 See, for example, Guenter B. Risse, R. L. Numbers, and J. W. Leavitt (eds.), *Medicine without Doctors: Home Health Care in American History* (New York: Science Publications, 1977).

9 Rosemary Stevens, *American Medicine and the Public Interest* (New Haven: Yale University Press, 1971), pp. 35–59.

10 Alex Berman, "Neo-Thomsonianism in the United States," *Journal of the History of Medicine*, 11 (1956), 133–155, presents these botanists in a rather unfavorable light.

11 Joseph F. Kett, *The Formation of the American Medical Profession: The Role of Institutions, 1780–1860* (New Haven: Yale University Press, 1968); Martin Kaufman, *Homeopathy in America: The Rise and Fall of a Medical Heresy* (Baltimore: Johns Hopkins Press, 1971).

12 See Charles Rosenberg's introduction to D. W. Cathell, *The Physician Himself and What He Should Add to His Scientific Acquirements* (1882; reprint ed.,

New York; ARNO Press, 1972); Duffy, *The Healers*, pp. 234–236; and George Rosen, *The Specialization of Medicine, with Particular Reference to Ophthalmology* (New York: Froben Press, 1944), pp. 62–64.

13 Duffy, *The Healers*, pp. 234–240.

14 See Rosen, *The Specialization of Medicine*, pp. 62–70, in which he points out that a strong interest in pecuniary rewards motivated some to specialize; see also Gerald Markowitz and David K. Rosner, "Doctors in Crisis: Medical Education and Medical Reform during the Progressive Era, 1895–1915," in Susan Reverby and David Rosner (eds.), *Health Care in America: Essays in Social History* (Philadelphia: Temple University Press, 1979), pp. 185–205.

15 Cathell, *The Physician Himself*, pp. 27–28; see also Arpad G. Gerster, *Recollections of a New York Surgeon* (New York: Paul B. Hoeber, 1917), pp. 23–24.

16 Cathell, *The Physician Himself*, p. 1.

17 Gerster, *Recollections*, p. 162.

18 Charles Rosenberg, "The Therapeutic Revolution: Medicine, Meaning, and Social Change in Nineteenth Century America," in Morris J. Vogel and Charles Rosenberg (eds.), *The Therapeutic Revolution: Essays in the Social History of American Medicine* (Philadelphia: University of Pennsylvania Press, 1979), pp. 3–25.

19 See, for example, Charles Rosenberg, *The Cholera Years* (Chicago: University of Chicago Press, 1962), for a discussion of moral notions of illness and the role of medical therapeutics.

20 There are a number of recent works on this subject. See Morris J. Vogel, *The Invention of the Modern Hospital: Boston, 1880–1930* (Chicago: University of Chicago Press, 1980); Charles Rosenberg, "Inward Vision and Outward Glance: The Shaping of the Modern Hospital, 1880–1914," *Bulletin of the History of Medicine*, 53 (Fall 1979), 346–391; and David Rosner, "Business at the Bedside: Health Care in Brooklyn, 1890–1915," in Reverby and Rosner, *Health Care in America*, pp. 117–131.

21 Chinese Hospital Association, *1st Annual Report*, 1892, p. 1.

22 See "Hospitals and Dispensaries," in Bureau of the Census, *Special Report on Benevolent Institutions* (Washington, D.C.: Government Printing Office, 1913), pp. 327–330, which lists the names, sizes, and founding dates of New York and Brooklyn hospitals and dispensaries.

23 Methodist Hospital, *9th Annual Report*, Nov. 1895–Oct. 1896, pp. 23–25.

24 Ibid., pp. 22–24.

25 See, for example, the picture of the building that the Lutheran Hospital occupied from 1884 to as late as the second decade of the twentieth century, in Lutheran Hospital Association, *Annual Report*, 1914, p. 2; also see the picture of old Bethany Hospital in its *12th Annual Report*, 1906, frontispiece; and see Chinese Hospital Association, *1st Annual Report*, 1892, p. 2. See also, Phillip Jacobs, *New Hospitals Needed in Greater New York*, State Charities Aid Association of New York, Publication No. 101 (New York: State Charities Aid Association of New York, 1908), p. 81: Ten of the eighteen church facilities listed in Jacobs's report had fewer than 100

beds. Some of the hospitals listed had as few as 18 beds, and none of the charity facilities had more than 321. The facility with 321 beds, St. Peters, devoted 20 percent of its work to consumptives.

26   Brooklyn Homeopathic Maternity, *Constitution, By-Laws and Regulations*, 1890, p. 17. See also Brooklyn Nursery and Infants' Hospital, *25th Annual Report*, 1896, p. 9, which says that the "work of the household shall be performed as far as possible by the mothers of children who are inmates"; and Brooklyn Home for Consumptives, *30th Annual Report*, Oct. 1911, pp. 63–64: "Those [patients] who are able will be expected to . . . render such service as they can for the benefit of the Institution and the comfort of those more helpless than themselves."

27   Chinese Hospital Association, *1st Annual Report*, 1892, p. 2.

28   Ibid.

29   See, for example, the description in ibid., pp. 1–2, of one patient who stayed in the hospital for 217 days although he had been "cured" of all illness. When he left, against the urgings of the trustees, he fell ill once more and returned to the hospital, where he died a "happy Christian."

30   Chinese Hospital Association, *1st Annual Report*, 1892, p. 3.

31   John Duffy, *A History of Public Health in New York City, 1886–1966*, vol. 2 (New York: Russell Sage Foundation, 1974).

32   Brooklyn Association for Improving the Conditions of the Poor, *46th Annual Report*, 1888, p. 13.

33   For a detailed discussion of the development of the suburban neighborhood and the effects of the electric trolley on urban growth see two books by Sam Bass Warner, Jr., *Streetcar Suburbs: The Process of Growth in Boston, 1870–1900* (New York: Atheneum, 1962), and *The Urban Wilderness: A History of the American City* (New York: Harper & Row, 1972).

34   David McCullogh, *The Great Bridge* (New York: Simon & Schuster, 1972).

35   Inter-Racial Council, "Distribution of the Foreign-born in New York City, 1919" (mimeo, New York City Municipal Library), gives an account of the locations, jobs, and significant cultural characteristics of the various immigrant groups that settled in New York and Brooklyn during the previous thirty years. Also see McCullogh, *The Great Bridge*, pp. 110–112, for a fine description of late-nineteenth-century Brooklyn.

36   See Census Office, Department of the Interior, *Report on Manufacturing Industries in the United States at the 11th Census: 1890*, pt. II, *Statistics of Cities* (Washington, D.C.: Government Printing Office, 1895), pp. 88–97, tab. 3; also see Harold C. Syrett, *The City of Brooklyn* (New York: Columbia University Press, 1944), pp. 1–20; and Bureau of the Census, *Special Reports – Occupations at the 12th Census, 1900* (Washington, D.C.: Government Printing Office, 1904), pp. 634–653.

37   Census Office, *Report on Manufacturing Industries*, pt. II, p. xxvii.

38   Bureau of the Census, *Earnings of Factory Workers, 1899–1927*, Census Monograph X (Washington, D.C.: Government Printing Office, 1929), pp. 300–302.

39   "What It Costs to Live," *NY Trib*, Nov. 19, 1906, p. 5.

40 Jacobs, *New Hospitals Needed,* p. 29.

41 Lewis Pilcher, "Changing Condition of Professional Work in the City of Brooklyn," *BMJ,* 1 (Jan. 1881), 1–2. Elsewhere, Pilcher remarked that Brooklyn was "somewhat dazed by the conditions that attend its rapid growth." See Pilcher, "Public Hospitals of Brooklyn," *BMJ,* 4 (Aug. 1890), 534–535.

42 See John A. Hornsby and Richard E. Schmidt, *The Modern Hospital: Its Inspiration, Its Architecture, Its Equipment, Its Operation* (Philadelphia: Saunders, 1913), p. 34.

43 Bushwick Hospital, *12th Annual Report,* Mar. 1905–Mar. 1906, p. 14. See also Memorial Hospital for Women and Children, *Annual Report,* 1892, p. 14: "We find ourselves again obliged to secure a larger building, in order to accommodate a greater number of patients."

44 See "Hospitals and Ambulances," *NYTrib,* July 21, 1902, p. 6: "Accidents have been frequent within the city limits this year. Subway excavation and blasting, the wounding and maiming of the victims of trolley. . . ." See also Phillip Jacobs, *Ambulance Service in Greater New York,* State Charities Aid Association of New York, Publication No. 99 (New York: State Charities Aid Association of New York, 1907), p. 14; and "Prospectus of the Brooklyn Throat Hospital," Nov. 1889, p. 10: "The hospital is placed in the centre of one of the largest manufacturing districts in the country, a district, too, where an unusually large proportion of the workmen, some by reason of constant exposure as in the freight yards, and some by confinement in hot atmospheres in sugar houses or foundries, are unusually prone to pulmonary troubles."

45 Methodist Hospital, *4th Annual Report,* 1891, p. 24. See also Jacobs, *Ambulance Service,* p. 15.

46 Jacobs, *Ambulance Service,* p. 26. See also "Dying Patients Jolted through Streets in Crowded Ambulances," *NYTrib,* Feb. 25, 1906, p. 1, for discussion of the need for hospital efficiency and ambulance service.

47 Jacobs, *New Hospitals Needed,* p. 25.

48 Ibid., pp. 57, 76.

49 See, for example, the obituary of Abraham Abraham, *NYT,* June 29, 1911, p. 11: "Mr. Abraham was a pioneer in the development of the big shopping district of Brooklyn . . . The business of [Abraham and Straus] cover[ed] about seven acres of land [by the time of his death]."

50 Brooklyn Eye and Ear Hospital, *38th Annual Report,* 1906, p. 4.

51 William Browning, "The New Home of Our Society," *BMJ,* 16 (Feb. 1902), 77–78.

52 Ibid.; see also George McNaughton, "Laying the Cornerstone of the New Building," *BMJ,* 16 (Feb. 1902), 53.

53 Memorial Hospital for Women and Children, *4th Annual Report,* 1895, pp. 19–20.

54 Bushwick and East Brooklyn Dispensary, *15th Annual Report,* May 1893, p. 9.

55 Brooklyn Homeopathic Maternity, *19th Annual Report,* 1889, p. 11. See also

Brooklyn Women's Homeopathic Hospital and Dispensary, *Annual Report*, 1888, p. 8: "Our present location on the line of the Fulton Street Elevated R.R. is no longer suitable." By 1891, the Brooklyn Homeopathic Maternity claimed that change of location was an "imperative necessity," because "the Bridge with its noise and bustle and its increasing traffic, has come up to us." See Brooklyn Homeopathic Maternity, *21st Annual Report*, 1891, p. 10.

56   The area known as Crown Heights has shifted southward over the years but still has Eastern Parkway as a major thoroughfare. Not until 1928 was the area finally urbanized. See "New Garden Apartment House Section Developing on Last of Crown Heights Vacant Land," *BDE*, Sept. 2, 1928: "What was known not many years ago as the Crown Heights, but which has now been merged into one homogeneous section known as the Eastern Parkway districts is undergoing the finishing operations which wipe out the last trace or vestige of vacant plots of any great size." See also *Brooklyn Communities – Population Characteristics and Neighborhood Social Resources* (New York: Bureau of Community Statistical Services, Research Department, Community Council of Greater New York, 1959), p. 98, which describes the Bedford area: "In the 1920's and in previous years much of the downtown or Bedford section of the community was a prosperous home-owning, middle-class neighborhood with . . . many one family brownstone or whitestone of the three or four floor . . . type."

For data on the housing boom in the Crown Heights–Bedford area, see "Brooklyn Real Estate Boom Spreading," *BDE*, Aug. 17, 1891, p. 4; "Brooklyn Real Estate Book Helped by Rapid Transit," *BDE*, July 6, 1891, p. 1; "Wyckoff and Livingston Farms Taken for Building Sites," *BDE*, July 27, 1891, p. 4; "Eastern Parkway, Brisk Sales," *BDE*, Apr. 19, 1892, p. 6; and "Good Price for Pacific Street Property," *BDE*, July 14, 1892, p. 1. For a more general view of suburbanization of the period, see Warner, *Streetcar Suburbs*.

57   Brooklyn Women's Homeopathic Hospital, *Annual Report*, 1888, p. 8.

58   W. H. Snyder and H. H. Morton, "Resolution," *Kings County Medical Society Monthly Bulletin*, Mar. 1910, n.p.; and James Fleming, W. H. Snyder, and H. H. Morton, "Letter," ibid., Mar. 1910, n.p. The authors of the "Resolution" discuss the problems of refurbishing a doctor's office: "Each specialist requires an elaborate outfit of apparatus for his work, and rooms especially arranged with reference to size and lighting . . . surgeons need a good light and a series of connecting rooms . . . Even if it were possible to buy or rent thirty or forty houses on the Heights, each house would require more or less expensive alterations and additions before it could serve the purpose of a doctor's office."

59   Snyder and Morton, "Resolution," n.p.; see also Fleming, Snyder, and Morton "Letter."

60   The introduction of the telephone into the private offices of physicians was rapid and facilitated communication with clients who were outside a

walking radius around the offices. In 1890, for instance, a sample of 215 Brooklyn physicians listed in the *Medical Register of New York, New Jersey, and Connecticut, 1889–90* (New York: Putnam, 1889), shows only 6 with telephone service. By 1918 a similar sample of 200 Brooklyn physicians shows only 6 *without* telephone service.

61 These data were derived from the following table:

	1890	1900	1910	1918
No. of physicians on three specified blocks in Brooklyn	206	423	639	727
No. of physicians in Brooklyn	1,215	1,742	2,172	2,500
Physicians on specified blocks as % of physicians in Brooklyn	16.9	24.3	29.4	29.1

Sources: "Street Lists of Brooklyn Physicians," *Medical Directories,* 1890, 1900, 1910, 1918; Bureau of the Census, Statistics on Population, pt. II, *11th Census, 1890* (Washington, D.C.: Government Printing Office, 1897), pp. 640–641, tab. 118; idem, *Special Reports – Occupations at the 12th Census* (Washington, D.C.: Government Printing Office, 1900); idem, *Population – Occupation Statistics for 13th Census* (Washington, D.C.: Government Printing Office, 1910), 4:580–581. Statistics for 1918 were approximated on the basis of census data for 1920 (Bureau of the Census, *Population – 14th Census* [Washington, D.C.: Government Printing Office, 1920], vol. 4).

62 Census Office, Department of the Interior, *Vital Statistics of New York City and Brooklyn, covering a Period of Six Years Ending May 31, 1890* (Washington, D.C.: Government Printing Office, 1894).

63 Ibid., pp. 185–188. This report gave the relative mortality and morbidity rates for each area of the city, as well as age-specific rates.

64 See ibid., pp. 218–225, for a description of the healthy conditions of most of the areas into which physicians were moving.

65 See Syrett, *City of Brooklyn,* p. 18, for early newspaper accounts of the miserable living conditions in the Navy Yard area. Also see McCullogh, *The Great Bridge,* p. 112: McCullogh notes that "the tenements on the 'flats' south of the Navy Yard, where a larger part of Brooklyn's Irish lived, were as foul as any in New York."

66 These data are drawn from the "Street Lists of Physicians," *Medical Directories,* 1890 and 1918. Though the number of physicians per 1,000 residents remained relatively stable, with the physician population for the city as a whole varying between 1.3 and 1.5 per 1,000 (see the following table), the number of physicians in the Navy Yard area was much lower – only 0.6 per 1,000 in 1890.

	1890	1900	1910	1920
No. of physicians in Brooklyn	1,213	1,742	2,172	2,704
Population of Brooklyn	806,343	1,166,582	1,634,354	2,018,356
No. of physicians per 1,000 residents	1.5	1.5	1.3	1.3

67 The migration of doctors away from poorer areas is a historical process that is still going on today. A modern study by the Department of Health in New York City showed that the area to which doctors moved during the Progressive era is now devoid of physicians. The once pastoral neighborhood around Lafayette Street has since become the heart of Bedford-Stuyvesant and, as the study shows, now has the fewest doctors of any area in the city. See "A Virtual Lack of Doctors Found in Some Slum Areas of New York," *NYT*, Dec. 13, 1977, p. 45.

2. Embattled benefactors

1 Sidney Lens, *The Labor Wars* (Garden City, N.Y.: Anchor, 1974), p. 93.
2 Lillian Wald, *The House on Henry Street* (New York: Dover, facsimile ed., 1971), p. 17.
3 Brooklyn Hospital, *Annual Report*, 1897, p. 7.
4 Methodist Hospital, *3rd Annual Report*, Nov. 1890, pp. 15–18. See also *Completing a Great Charity, The Methodist General Hospital: Its Origin, Purposes, Needs* (New York, 1887), pp. 1–2, in which the hospital requests donations: "To complete these buildings and support the seventy-five beds . . . *the reader of this pamphlet is invited to contribute.*"
5 Brooklyn Throat Hospital, *Prospectus*, Nov. 1889, p. 11.
6 Long Island Throat and Lung Hospital, *3rd Annual Report*, 1892, p. 7. Similar themes had been used in almost all nineteenth-century facilities. In the Lucretia Mott Dispensary, Infirmary and Hospital, for instance, deficits and costs for new construction had been closely linked: "[The Dispensary] has [functioned] only through the kind assistance of a few, a very few, of the charitable people of Brooklyn; and on this account the means and accommodations of the Institution are far more limited in scope and plan of its work . . . To enable us to [expand our work] we need pecuniary aid, and it is our purpose at the present time to show why charitable people . . . should help us with a liberal hand." See the Lucretia Mott Dispensary and Infirmary, *A Brief General Review of Its Work* (New York, 1894), p. 6.
7 Frederick Sturges, "What Managers of the Hospital Say about Their Financial Problem," *Charities*, 12 (Jan. 2, 1904), 32.

8   Memorial Hospital for Women and Children, "A Few Words" (circular), p. 1–3.
9   Memorial Hospital for Women and Children, *10th Annual Report*, 1898, p. 16.
10 "Curtailment of Hospital Work Threatens New York," *Charities*, 12 (Jan. 9, 1904), 65.
11 Methodist Hospital, *7th Annual Report*, 1894, p. 19.
12 Brooklyn Maternity, *26th Annual Report*, 1896, p. 11.
13 Brooklyn Eye and Ear Hospital, *31st Annual Report*, 1899, pp. 1–2.
14 Brooklyn Nursery and Infants' Hospital, *25th Annual Report*, 1896, p. 15. See also Methodist Hospital, *8th Annual Report*, 1895, p. 15: "We were confronted at the outset by the certainty that our expenses would be . . . in excess . . . More beds were in use, and more patients would therefore be treated."
15 Brooklyn Eye and Ear Hospital, *30th Annual Report*, 1898, p. 4. In 1896 the directors also noted that "the sources of revenue from individual subscriptions are diminishing . . . The *legacies* to the hospital have been few in number." See idem, *28th Annual Report*, 1896, p. 3; Brooklyn Central Throat Hospital, *Annual Reports*, 1893–1897; Brooklyn Maternity Hospital, *Annual Reports*, 1893–1894; and Brooklyn Memorial Hospital for Women and Children, *Annual Reports*, 1892–1898.
16 Brooklyn Hospital, *Annual Report*, 1895, p. 6.
17 Editorial, *Trained Nurse and Hospital Review*, 29 (Sept. 1902), 194. See also Brooklyn Hospital, *Annual Report*, 1899, p. 8: "Deficits of recent years [have] resulted in a floating debt [of] about twenty-seven thousand dollars."
18 New York Hospital (NYH), *Board of Governors, Minutes*, Mar. 5, 1901, p. 147, in NYH Archives. (All references regarding NYH refer to materials in the archives unless otherwise noted.)
19 Brooklyn Central Dispensary and Hospital, *Annual Report*, Jan. 1895, pp. 7–8. See also Charity Organization Society of New York, *Annual Report*, July 1899–June 1900, p. 19: "Several of the large private hospitals are having increased difficulty in securing from private subscriptions each year the funds necessary to meet their current expenses."
20 Brooklyn Eye and Ear Hospital, *28th Annual Report*, 1896, p. 3.
21 Brooklyn Eye and Ear Hospital, *30th Annual Report*, 1898, p. 3.
22 Brooklyn Hospital, *Annual Report*, 1903, p. 7. See also Bedford Dispensary and Hospital, *Annual Report*, 1897, p. 9: "Our hospital facilities have been increased to four beds"; Memorial Hospital for Women and Children, *4th Annual Report*, 1892, p. 14: "At the close of the year we find ourselves again obligated to secure a larger building, in order to accommodate a greater number of patients"; and Bushwick Hospital, *12th Annual Report*, March 1905–1906, p. 15: "With the population and business rapidly increasing . . . the demands made upon our hospital will be proportionately enlarged, and our present capacity is now being taxed to its utmost. The need for a larger and better equipped building is imperative."

23   NYH, *Board of Governors Minutes*, Mar. 5, 1901, p. 147.
24   Frank Tucker, "The Hospital Situation in New York's Hospitals," *Charities*, 12 (Jan. 2, 1904), 27. See also Methodist Hospital, *7th Annual Report*, 1894, p. 18.
25   Methodist Hospital, *7th Annual Report*, 1894, p. 18.
26   "A Hospital Conference in New York," *Charities*, 13 (Mar. 11, 1905), 565.
27   "Curtailment of Hospital Work Menaces New York," p. 65.
28   Brooklyn Hospital, *Annual Report*, 1893, p. 9.
29   See Brooklyn Maternity, *25th Annual Report*, 1895, p. 14, for an itemized list of the functions that netted small sums for the institution.
30   Editorial, "Hospital Debts," *Trained Nurse and Hospital Review*, 14 (Mar. 1895), 161. See also the *Annual Reports* for other years for examples of the varied functions that lent support to the Maternity. Nearly all of the city's hospitals engaged in extended efforts to increase charitable donations.
31   Bushwick [Central] Hospital, *10th Annual Report*, Mar. 1903–1904, p. 12. See also Bushwick and Bushwick Central Hospital, *11th Annual Report*, Mar. 1904–1905, p. 12; and Bushwick Hospital, *13th Annual Report*, Mar. 1906–1907, p. 11.
32   See Brooklyn Hospital, *Annual Report*, 1904, p. 8, for one example: "Edward H. Kidder [resignation] made necessary by his removal from Brooklyn."
33   Bushwick and Bushwick Central Hospital, *11th Annual Report*, Mar. 1904–1905, p. 12. See also the obituary of H. C. Bohack, *NYT*, Sept. 18, 1931, p. 23: "President of Bohack Chain of 746 stores . . . H. C. Bohack was born in Germany in 1865, opened his first store in 1885." He had five stores by 1900, and was president of a realty corporation and director of People's National Bank, Guarantee Title and Mortgage Co., Brooklyn National Life Insurance Co., Hamburg Savings Bank, and Manhattan Trust.
34   For a brief synopsis of the Pratt family history in Brooklyn see *Dictionary of American Biography*, s.v. "Pratt, Charles." See also the obituary of Abraham Abraham, *NYT*, June 29, 1911, p. 11: "Mr. Abraham was a pioneer in the development of the big shopping district in Brooklyn. [It covered] about 7 acres of land . . . indicating the importance of the man in commercial Brooklyn."
35   Though I have cast the primary issue dividing trustees in terms of income source and economic position, Hofstadter recognizes a similar trend in the larger society and relates this process to the age of particular persons promoting reform. "During the next twenty years [after 1890] the dominant new influence came from those who were still young enough to have their thinking affected by the hard problems just emerging, problems for which the older generation . . . had no precedents and no convincing answers" (Richard Hofstadter, *Age of Reform* [New York: Vintage, 1955], p. 166).
36   Brooklyn Eastern District Dispensary and Hospital, *13th Annual Report*, 1891, pp. 7–8.
37   Lutheran Hospital Association, *Annual Report*, 1914, p. 21.
38   Jewish Hospital, *2nd Annual Report*, 1903, p. 10.

39 Frank Tucker, "The Public Conscience and the Hospital," *Charities*, 13 (Dec. 13, 1904), 285; W. Emlen Roosevelt, "Response to Tucker's 'Hospital Situation in New York,' " *Charities*, 12 (Jan. 2, 1904), 37.

40 Tucker, "Hospital Situation in New York," p. 31.

41 Sturges, "What the Managers of the Hospital Say," p. 32. Sturges also pointed out (p. 34) that "the founders and the charter members of the great private hospitals, and their direct descendants, are the ones who are now principally carrying them, and it is extremely difficult to interest the younger generation."

42 Governors of NYH, "Report of the Committee on Finance and Retrenchment," *Minutes*, Mar. 5, 1901, p. 174.

43 NYH, *Papers*, 1905–1906, folder 2: 1905 finance committee, for "List of Investments."

44 See Henry C. Crane, "History of the Society of New York Hospital, 1769–1920" (microfilm, NYH Archives), p. 391a.

45 See Society of NYH, *Minutes*, Mar. 5, 1901, p. 147; see also NYH, *Treasurer Papers*, 1901–1902, folder 1: 1902 Fiscal Committee on Finance and Retrenchment, pp. 5–8.

46 Society of NYH, *Minutes*, Apr. 7, 1903, pp. 306–307.

47 Jewish Hospital, *2nd Annual Report*, 1903, p. 8; Memorial Hospital for Women and Children, *10th Annual Report*, 1898, p. 18; Sturges, "What the Managers of the Hospitals Say," p. 32.

48 "Homeopathic Hospital to Close This Evening," *BDE*, Mar. 31, 1900. See also "Williamsburg Hospital Closes," *NYTrib*, Jan. 16, 1901; "City Takes the Hospital," *BDE*, July 26, 1900; "Hospital Bill Hearing To-day," *BDE*, Mar. 7, 1900; and "Anent the Homeopaths," *BDE*, Mar. 6, 1900.

49 Brooklyn Nursery and Infants' Hospital, *23rd Annual Report*, 1893–1894, pp. 15–16.

50 Methodist Hospital, *8th Annual Report*, 1895, p. 22.

51 Methodist Hospital, *13th Annual Report*, 1900, p. 14; see also the hospital's annual reports from 1894 to 1897.

52 For data on declining length of patient stays, see Methodist Hospital, *Annual Reports*, 1894–1900 (specifically, 1895, p. 12, and 1900, p. 14); and Brooklyn Hospital, *Annual Reports*, 1885–1915.

53 Memorial Hospital for Women and Children, *10th Annual Report*, 1898, p. 18.

54 Brooklyn Eastern District Dispensary and Hospital, *Annual Report*, 1891, p. 8.

55 Brooklyn Hospital, *Annual Report*, 1899, p. 8.

56 Ibid., 1900, p. 7.

57 Editorial Comment, *Trained Nurse and Hospital Review*, 29 (Sept. 1902), 194.

58 Methodist Hospital, *3rd Annual Report*, 1890, p. 16.

59 Lutheran Hospital Association, *Annual Report*, 1914, p. 21.

60 Methodist Hospital, *7th Annual Report*, 1894, p. 20. Also see Long Island College Hospital (LICH), *Hospital Yearbook*, 1919, p. 35, for a later statement of the increasing pressure to get paying patients into the hospital.

61   A. C. Bunn, "Church Hospitals," *BMJ*, 15 (Sept. 1901), 508.
62   Jewish Hospital, *2nd Annual Report*, Nov. 1903, p. 11.
63   Lutheran Hospital Association, *Annual Report*, 1914, p. 2. See also Brooklyn
     Homeopathic Maternity, *19th Annual Report*, 1889, p. 12, where the secre-
     tary disdainfully notes that "other maternities in this and our sister city . . .
     demand pay for every patient [whereas] we work largely for charity."
64   Bushwick Hospital, *13th Annual Report*, 1906–1907, p. 15.
65   Ogden Chisholm, "Financial Problems of New York's Hospitals," *Charities*,
     12 (June 2, 1904), 38.
66   See Robert L. Dickinson, "Hospital Organization As Shown by Charts of
     Personnel and Powers Functions," *Bulletin of the Taylor Society*, 3 (Oct. 1917),
     1–11. I am indebted to Susan Reverby of Boston University for pointing
     out this article. Among persons who listened to and commented on Dickin-
     son's paper were Ernest Codman, the well-known Boston surgeon and
     hospital rationalizer who formulated the "End-Result" system in hospital
     work, and Frank Gilbreth, the prominent exponent of Taylorism in facto-
     ry work. Nurses and hospital superintendents were also present for the
     reading of Dickinson's paper.
67   Ernest Codman, Response to "Dickinson's 'Hospital Organization . . . ,' "
     Bulletin of the Taylor Society, 3 (Oct. 1917), 6. Codman, a controversial advo-
     cate of standardization in surgery, felt that the vision of a "charity" hospi-
     tal was hypocritical. He wanted the cloak of charity pulled away and the
     standardized, "scientific" hospital developed. Ironically, at the very height
     of the "scientific medicine" movement, Codman was ostracized for his
     views by his colleagues at Massachusetts General Hospital and was forced
     to leave that institution. See Susan Reverby, "Stealing the Golden Eggs:
     Ernest Amory Codman and the Science and Management of Medicine,"
     Bulletin of the History of Medicine, 55 (Summer 1981), 156–171, for a fascinat-
     ing account of the conflict among practitioners over the goals of medicine.

3.   Social class and hospital care

1   Frank Tucker, "The Hospital Situation in New York's Hospitals," *Charities*,
     12 (Jan. 2, 1904), 30. See also A. C. Bunn, "Church Hospitals," *BMJ*, 15
     (Sept. 1901), 510. See also Charlotte Aikens, "Relation of the Training
     School to the Hospital Deficit Problem," *Trained Nurse and Hospital Review*, 37
     (Sept. 1910), 157: "The extension and improvement of the pay patient
     departments . . . is one of the remedies for deficits that is meeting with
     general favor."
2   Homer Folks, Comment on Frank Tucker, "The Financial Problems of
     New York's Hospitals," *Charities*, 12 (Jan. 2, 1904), 46.
3   Jesse T. Duryea, "City versus Independent Hospitals," *BMJ*, 15 (Sept.
     1901), 496. See also "Scope and Support of City Hospitals," *BDE*, Mar. 20,
     1901, in DSML clippings, in which Duryea is quoted as follows: "A large
     number of cases inspected by our examiners were found to be able to pay
     at least the minimum rate."

4 Sidney Goldstein, "Social Function of the Hospital," *Charities*, 18 (May 4, 1907), 162. Also see remarks on the difficulty of identifying the social class of patients in Editorial, "Abuse of Medical Charity," *Trained Nurse and Hospital Review*, 19 (Aug. 1897), 101.

5 T. J. Hillis, "Hospital Mismanagement," *Medical News* (New York), 79 (Nov. 9, 1901), 722–723.

6 Editorial, "Public Hospital or Private Sanitarium," *Trained Nurse and Hospital Review*, 18 (Jan. 1897), 44.

7 Editorial, "Abolish the Hospital Grafter," *Journal of the American Medical Association* (*JAMA*), 44 (May 27, 1905), p. 1691.

8 Editorial, "The Problems of the Hospitals," *NYT*, Jan. 26, 1904, p. 8. Others in Manhattan also recognized that changing housing patterns of the city had promoted the use of the hospital. See, for instance, Tucker, "Hospital Situation in New York," p. 30; and editorial, "Private Sanitarium," *BMJ*, 2 (Apr. 1893), 219, in which the editors point out that hotels and apartments increased the need for new types of boardinghouse health care. Morris J. Vogel's interesting volume also illustrates this point for Boston: See *The Invention of the Modern Hospital: Boston, 1870–1930* (Chicago: University of Chicago Press, 1980).

9 Editorial, "The Problems of the Hospitals," p. 8.

10 Ibid.

11 Ibid.

12 F. R. Sturgis, "Other Views of New York Hospitals and Their Annual Deficits," *Charities*, 12 (Jan. 30, 1904), 112–113.

13 Ibid., p. 112.

14 "The Hospital Superintendents on the Hospital Situation in New York," *Charities*, 12 (Feb. 6, 1904), 157–158.

15 Ibid., pp. 158–161.

16 Ibid., p. 158.

17 Ibid., p. 159. There was a debate over whether private patient fees should be seen as a significant source of income. See John Harrigan, "The Advantage to the Public and the City of the Non-Municipal Hospital," *BMJ*, 15 (Sept. 1901), 505: "Reference has been made to the practice that obtains in non-municipal hospitals of devoting the profits that are realized from . . . full pay or private room patients to . . . helping to defray the expense . . . of non-pay patients"; Franklin A. Cleveland, "The Advantages of Accurate and Coordinated Statistics in Hospitals," *Charities*, 15 (Nov. 18, 1905), 251: "The theory is that private patients should be taken only at a profit"; John A. Hornsby and Richard E. Schmidt, *The Modern Hospital: Its Inspiration, Its Architecture, Its Equipment, Its Operation* (Philadelphia: Saunders, 1913), p. 21; Bushwick Hospital, *14th Annual Report*, Mar. 1907–Mar. 1908, p. 12; Brooklyn Hospital, *Annual Report*, 1898, p. 6; and Stephen Smith, "Report of Commission on Hospitals: 2nd NYS Conference of Charities and Correction," *Charities*, 7 (Nov. 30, 1901), 469.

18 "Hospital Superintendents on the Hospital Situation in New York," p. 160.

19 Ibid., pp. 160–161. Fisher, superintendent at Presbyterian Hospital, saw

"no reason why those who are treated free, and those who pay the nominal sum . . . should not be treated under precisely the same conditions and in the same buildings and wards. Those who pay for private services and for luxuries should be distinctly separated from the general free service." Noted Glover: "I see no reason whatever why there should be any division between patients who pay nothing and those who can pay something." Hiram Calkins, president of Hahnemann Hospital, had a slightly different viewpoint: He did "not approve either Dr. Sturgis' or the *New York Times* classification of patients [or] the placing of each class in separate buildings," because both "are impracticable and would prove to be detrimental to the best care of the patient" (ibid., p. 163).

20 Harrigan, "Advantage to the Public," p. 505.
21 Cleveland, "Advantages of Accurate and Coordinated Statistics," p. 251. See also "New York Hospitals," *Charities*, 6 (Jan. 5, 1901), p. 4: "In private rooms there is paid something more than the cost, and . . . we obtain a certain income for the benevolent work in the wards"; and John Brown and Edward Fletcher, "A General Hospital for One Hundred Patients," in Aikens (ed.), *Hospital Management: A Handbook for Hospital Trustees, Superintendents, Training School Principals, Physicians and All Others Actively Engaged in Promoting Hospital Work* (Philadelphia: Saunders, 1911), p. 125: "The profits . . . are applied [to the charity facilities]."
22 Hornsby and Schmidt, *The Modern Hospital*, p. 19.
23 President's Statement, Brooklyn Hospital, *Annual Report*, 1896, p. 6.
24 NYH, *Secretary-Treasurer's Papers*, 1901–1902, folders: 1901 Visiting Committee, Report to Committee from Various Persons; and 1901 Real Estate, Leases, Bills, Receipts.
25 Ibid.
26 Brooklyn Hospital, *Minutes*, 4 (Oct. 25, 1894), p. 242.
27 Ibid., 4 (Sept. 28, 1893), p. 179.
28 Ibid., 4 (Dec. 3, 1894), n.p.
29 William Hollenback Cary, "Brooklyn Hospital," *LIMJ*, 4 (Oct. 1910), p. 356.
30 See, for example, street maps and *BDE* articles of the period that refer to Brooklyn Hospital as the "City Hospital."
31 William Low, "Presidential Message," Brooklyn Hospital, *Annual Report*, 1892, p. 4.
32 Brooklyn Hospital, *Minutes*, 4 (Dec. 3, 1894), n.p.
33 Ibid.
34 Ibid.
35 See, for an example of the earlier ads, "Brooklyn Hospital," *BDE*, Jan. 5, 1895, p. 6.
36 See "Brooklyn Hospital," *BDE*, May 8, 1895, p. 6, for an example of later advertisements.
37 NYH, *Papers*, 1901–1902, folder 1: 1901 Real Estate Leases, Bills, Receipts, Roosevelt and NYH cards; and folder: 1901 Visiting Committee Reports, p. 3.

38   Editorial, "Bellevue Scandal," *NYT*, Dec. 31, 1900, p. 6.
39   Ibid., see also "New York Hospitals," *Charities*, p. 4: "It is sensible . . . to use [hospitals] rather than to attempt to treat patients at home."
40   NYC Department of Public Charities, "No Patients in Beds," in vertical file, New York City Department of Health, Public Health Library, New York City Hospital History.
41   "The Kings County Hospital," *BDE*, Jan. 12, 1895, p. 3; one patient quoted in the article maintained that these statements were false.
42   Ibid., p. 3.
43   "Seney Hospital Criticized," *NYT*, July 18, 1897, p. 19.
44   "In a Modern Hospital," *NYT*, Dec. 6, 1896, p. 13.
45   "Girl's Hospital Experience," *NYT*, June 4, 1899, p. 3.
46   Ibid.
47   "New York Hospitals," *NYT*, Dec. 31, 1900, p. 12; see this article for similar descriptions from other superintendents.
48   "Hospital Experience," p. 3.
49   "New York Hospitals," *NYT*, Dec. 31, 1900, p. 12.
50   "Hospital Experience," p. 3.
51   See, for example, "Girl's Hospital Experience," p. 3; "New York Hospitals," *NYT*, p. 12; "In a Modern Hospital," p. 16. Also see Susan Reverby's Ph.D. dissertation (" 'Apprenticeship to Duty': The Rationalization of American Nursing, 1860–1940," Boston University, 1982) on hospital and private-duty nursing.
52   "In a Modern Hospital," p. 16.
53   "Girl's Hospital Experience," p. 3.
54   "New York Hospitals," *NYT*, p. 12. The superintendent at Roosevelt Hospital, however, saw little problem with friends and relatives taking rooms in the hospital. One patient brought her husband and another companion, who took a room adjacent to hers.
55   See Brooklyn Hospital, *Annual Reports*, 1892–1915, for this financial data. The hospital reports give breakdowns for the amount of income derived from "free," "pay," and "private" patients for these years.
56   See Thomas Kessner, *The Golden Door* (New York: Oxford University Press, 1977).
57   Other comparisons also confirm that the hospital's shift to serving white-collar populations followed, rather than led, a general change in the city's class structure. For instance, see Table 5, which indicates that the working class still made up a significant proportion of the hospital's patients, although there was a substantial growth in the percentage of low-level white-collar jobs in the city during the period.
58   See Kessner, *The Golden Door*, pp. 181–184, for the occupational distribution of the Jewish population, and pp. 44–70 for a detailed discussion of occupational distinctions among Jews and Italians.
59   The sample of medical and surgical patients at the Jewish Hospital is similar to a sample drawn from information on birth certificates. The fathers of newborns also were about 30 percent white-collar and 70

percent blue-collar workers between 1907 and 1917.
60 These data are exclusive of those patients whose occupations are not listed in Table 7 (see the table footnote).
61 Tucker, "Hospital Situation in New York," p. 30.

4. Conflict in the new hospital

1 Brooklyn Hospital, *Minutes*, 4 (May 31, 1894), p. 233.
2 Ibid., 5 (Jan. 23, 1901), pp. 103–104.
3 Ibid., p. 104.
4 Ibid., 5 (Feb. 15, 1900), p. 66.
5 Ibid., 5 (Feb. 19, 1903), p. 203.
6 Ibid., 5 (Mar. 19, 1903), p. 200.
7 Ibid., 5 (Dec. 17, 1903), pp. 242–243; Brooklyn Hospital, *Annual Report*, 1900, pp. 6–7.
8 NYH, Letter to the Visiting Committee, Sept. 27, 1907, in *Papers*, folder: 1901 Visiting Committee Reports . . . from Various Persons.
9 See Rosemary Stevens, *American Medicine and the Public Interest* (New Haven: Yale University Press, 1971), for a description of the doctor's growing interest in specialism and clinical experiences; see also Gerald E. Markowitz and David K. Rosner, "Doctors in Crisis: Medical Education and Medical Reform during the Progressive Era, 1895–1915," in Susan Reverby and David Rosner (eds.), *Health Care in America: Essays in Social History* (Philadelphia: Temple University Press, 1979); and David Rosner, "Professional Interests and Patient Care: The Case of the Free-Standing Dispensary," *International Journal of Health Service Research*, forthcoming.
10 S. W. Hemphill to J. Raymond, Feb. 23, 1900, in files, DSML.
11 Martin Kaufman, *American Medical Education: The Formative Years, 1765–1910* (Westport, Conn.: Greenwood Press, 1976), pp. 144–146. There is an immense literature on nineteenth-century American medical education. See, for example, Kaufman, *American Medical Education*; and William F. Norwood, *Medical Education in the United States before the Civil War* (Philadelphia: University of Pennsylvania Press, 1944). For discussions of changes during the 1890s and after, see Markowitz and Rosner, "Doctors in Crisis." See E. Richard Brown, *Rockefeller Medicine Men: Medicine and Capitalism in America* (Berkeley and Los Angeles: University of California Press, 1979), for a more critical appraisal.
12 Henry R. Sanford to Joseph H. Raymond, May 12, 1899, in LICH files, DSML. Also see Sanford to Raymond, May 15, 1899, in LICH files, in which Sanford writes that his "State work takes me into every county of the State . . . bringing me into contact with teachers in great numbers, and I hope that my good opinion of the Long Island College Hospital will not be destroyed."
13 H. R. Sanford to J. H. Raymond, May 18, 1899, in LICH files, DSML. Although he was informed that James had failed six subjects, Sanford still

maintained that James could make up these subjects over the summer: "I understand that you have granted to some a condition of graduating in September next . . . Will you grant this for James? Does it seem fair to compel him to take another year?"

14 Lester D. Volk, "The Hospital Parasite and the Profession," *Medical Economist*, 3 (June 1915), 129.

15 Ibid.

16 L. D. Volk, "The Hospital Question," *Medical Economist*, 3 (Nov. 1915), 286–287; see also idem, "Old Abuses and New Monopolies," ibid., 3 (Oct. 1915), 252; "The Case of Dr. Dixon," ibid., 2 (Jan. 1914), 4–6; "The Hospital Question: A Tentative Solution," 3 (Sept. 1915), 201; L. D. Volk, "Our Hospital 'Open Door Policy' – Its Effect," ibid., 3 (Aug. 1915), 177.

17 Lewis Stephen Pilcher, "Professional Responsibility for Faulty Hospital Organization," *LIMJ*, 6 (Dec. 1912), 462.

18 Brooklyn Hospital, *Minutes*, 5 (Jan. 18, 1907), p. 386; ibid., 6 (Mar. 19, 1914), p. 301; ibid., 6 (Feb. 17, 1916), pp. 433, 444; Brooklyn Hospital, *Minutes of Executive Committee*, Mar. 11, 1916, p. 53.

19 Jewish Hospital, *2nd Annual Report*, Nov. 1903, p. 11.

20 NYH, *Papers*, 1901–1902, folder: 1901 Visiting Committee Reports . . . from Various Persons, Report of George Ludlam.

21 "Couldn't Bide Fishballs," *NYT*, Oct. 14, 1896, p. 9.

22 "Doctors Deposed from Office," *NYT*, Mar. 11, 1896, p. 10.

23 "Doctors Object to the Rules," *NYT*, Jan. 20, 1894, p. 9.

24 "St. John's Brooklyn Resignation," *NYTrib*, May 7, 1897, p. 4.

25 "German Hospital Staff Resigns – Physicians Leave Because Head Nurse Interfered with Their Work," *NYTrib*, Nov. 8, 1906, p. 10. See also "All Physicians Must Go – New Staff for the Homeopathic Hospital," *NYT*, Jan. 17, 1894, p. 9, for the statement that the board fired the entire staff because of "lack of unity and harmony," a charge denied, in turn, by the physicians; "To Establish a New Hospital," *NYTrib*, Feb. 6, 1894, p. 12, for the threat of the fired physicians to open up their own institution; and "No Revolution in the Board," *NYTrib*, Dec. 4, 1895, p. 5, for the reelection of those trustees who were in major part responsible for the firings, and hence the reaffirmation of trustees' right to govern the hospital.

26 Brooklyn Hospital, *Minutes*, 4 (May 25, 1893), 166–167.

27 Ibid., 4 (Mar. 28, 1895), n.p.

28 Ibid.

29 See Charles Rosenberg, "And Heal the Sick: The Hospital and Patient in Nineteenth Century America," *Journal of Social History*, 10 (June 1977), 428–447; and Morris J. Vogel, *The Invention of the Modern Hospital: Boston, 1870–1930* (Chicago: University of Chicago Press, 1980).

30 Methodist Hospital, *Exec. Comm. Minutes*, Nov. 8, 1892, pp. 181–182; ibid., Dec. 18, 1907, p. 63.

31 Letter to Surgeons and Physicians, p. 1, attached to Methodist Hospital, *Exec. Comm. Minutes*, Mar. 1, 1906, p. 67.

32 Ibid., see also, Methodist Hospital, *Exec. Comm. Minutes*, Apr. 20, 1897, for earlier statement.
33 Methodist Hospital, *Exec. Comm. Minutes*, Feb. 5, 1908, p. 73.
34 Ibid., June 9, 1908, p. 79.
35 Heber Hoople, "Economics of the Practice of Medicine," *BMJ*, 17 (June 1903), 270.
36 "Surgeon Sues Patients to Uphold a Principle," *BDE*, May 21, 1902, p. 1.
37 "Dr. Fowler Wins One Case," *BDE*, May 22, 1902, p. 1.
38 "Notice," *Charities*, 8 (May 31, 1902), 488.
39 Ibid.; see also "Physician and Hospitals Suffer Much from Deadbeats," *BDE*, June 1, 1902, p. 2.
40 "Dr. Fowler Wins Suit; Patients Must Pay Up," *BDE*, June 3, 1902, p. 2.
41 Ibid., p. 2.
42 See Rosenberg, "And Heal the Sick"; and Vogel, *Invention of the Modern Hospital*.
43 Report of Superintendent Kavanagh to Trustees, p. 3, attached to Methodist Hospital, *Exec. Comm. Minutes*, June 3, 1914, p. 221.
44 Ibid.
45 Ibid. See also letter from Walter T. Pilgrim (assistant superintendent to Kavanagh), back cover envelope, Methodist Hospital, *Exec. Comm. Minutes*, May 30, 1914: In reference to the problem of inappropriate accommodations, Pilgrim suggests that the board of managers "also take up the question of one of the principal causes of it, i.e. 'getting a patient in through pressure' when we are already taxed to our utmost. Often the patient and his friends become disgusted with the accommodation and then sign a release and complain of their treatment, when every effort has been made first to keep *them out* and then to keep *them in*." And see Methodist Hospital, *Board of Managers Minutes*, Sept. 26, 1907, p. 324.
46 Report of Kavanagh to Trustees, p. 3, attached to Methodist Hospital, *Exec. Comm. Minutes*, June 3, 1914, p. 221.
47 The numerous articles on the reasons for attaining hospital appointments often centered on these points. The *Medical Economist*, a New York City area journal published during this period by practitioners not associated with any particular hospital, was the most vocal and persistent observer of the economic interests of a hospital appointment.
48 Report of Kavanagh to Trustees, p. 1, attached to Methodist Hospital, *Exec. Comm. Minutes*, June 3, 1914, p. 221.
49 Ibid., p. 2.
50 See Markowitz and Rosner, "Doctors in Crisis"; and Stevens, *American Medicine*, pp. 80–97, for discussion of the oversupply of physicians and its effect on professional relationships.
51 See Stevens, *American Medicine*, pp. 77–171, for a fascinating account of the move toward specialization in medicine.
52 See Markowitz and Rosner, "Doctors in Crisis"; and Stevens, *American Medicine*, pp. 80–92, for discussions of competition among practitioners

and the development of the specialties, especially surgery.

53 See Stevens, *American Medicine*, p. 79, for a brief description.

54 Henry H. Morton to J. H. Raymond, Mar. 10, 1900, in LICH files, DSML.

55 Statement of Morton [to the Board of Regents], ca. May 1900, in LICH files, DSML, p. 4.

56 Ibid., p. 3–4.

57 Ibid.

58 H. H. Morton, "Presentation No. 1 in Regard to Seat in Hospital Facility," ca. June 1900, in LICH files, DSML, p. 4.

59 Editorial, "Is Genito Urinary Surgery a Specialty?" *Philadelphia Medical Journal*, May 12, 1900, as quoted in Morton, "Presentation No. 1," pp. 4–5.

60 See Letter to Board of Managers from the Surgical Staff, pp. 1–4, attached to Methodist Hospital, *Exec. Comm. Minutes*, Dec. 18, 1914, p. 261.

61 "Superintendent's Report," p. 2, attached to Methodist Hospital, *Exec. Comm. Minutes*, Dec. 20, 1914, p. 263.

62 "Superintendent's Reply," p. 1, attached to Methodist Hospital, *Exec. Comm. Minutes*, Dec. 18, 1914, p. 263.

63 Ibid., p. 6, attached to p. 261.

64 Report of Kavanagh to Trustees, p. 1, attached to Methodist Hospital, *Exec. Comm. Minutes*, June 3, 1914, p. 221.

65 "Superintendent's Observations," p. 3, attached to Methodist Hospital, *Exec. Comm. Minutes*, Dec. 20, 1914, p. 263.

66 Ibid. Doctors had tried to counter this argument by saying that the most famous surgeon, "when he began to operate at the founding of the Hospital, had but little experience"; to this one hospital trustee replied that those "were embryonic days, and that such standards would not suffice for the present development of the hospital" (ibid., p. 4).

67 Letter from the Medical Board to Trustees, pp. 3–4, attached to Methodist Hospital, *Exec. Comm. Minutes*, Dec. 18, 1914, p. 261.

68 See Methodist Hospital, *Exec. Comm. Minutes*, June 16, 1919, p. 55: "The question of Doctors collecting fees from paying ward patients brought in by themselves was discussed . . . [The by-laws were] amended . . . so as to read: '*The Attending physicians* and surgeons shall receive no compensation from patients treated in the wards of the Hospital . . . except with the knowledge and written consent of the Superintendent.' " See also "Charges to Patients," Methodist Hospital, *Exec. Comm. Minutes*, Apr. 20, 1897.

69 Methodist Hospital, *Exec. Comm. Minutes*, Dec. 20, 1914, p. 4, attachment to p. 163; ibid., July 23, 1915, p. 27; ibid., Jan. 27, 1915, p. 5.

70 Ibid., Feb. 1, 1915, p. 7.

71 See ibid., Mar. 18, 1915, p. 9, for quotation from Section 8 of the By-Laws of the Medical Board, adopted Dec. 2, 1914.

72 Letter to Secretary of Medical Board from Secretary of Board of Managers, Methodist Hospital, *Exec. Comm. Minutes*, Mar. 18, 1915, p. 1.

73 Methodist Hospital, *Exec. Comm. Minutes*, Dec. 20, 1914, p. 2, attachment to p. 263.

5. Taking control

1 William L. Riordan, *Plunkitt of Tammany Hall: A Series of Very Plain Talks on Very Practical Politics* (New York: Dutton, 1963), pp. 25–28. See also the interesting introduction by Arthur Mann.

2 Riordan, *Plunkitt of Tammany Hall*, pp. 27–28.

3 See Harold C. Syrett, *The City of Brooklyn* (New York: Columbia University Press, 1944), pp. 70–86, for a description of the local bosses who controlled patronage in Brooklyn during the second half of the nineteenth century. Syrett's description emphasizes the corruption of the bosses, but it should be remembered that local patronage has more recently been seen to be a rational mechanism of large nineteenth-century cities for provision of needed local services in the absence of a communication and transportation system. See Seymour J. Mandelbaum, *Boss Tweed's New York* (New York: Wiley, 1965), for a discussion of New York's response to rapid growth.

4 As early as 1890 there was a great concern for the future relationship between the city and charity health facilities. See Lewis Pilcher, "Public Hospitals of Brooklyn," *BMJ*, 4 (Aug. 1890), 539–541: "There has grown up in our city a peculiar state of affairs as regards the relations of the public treasury to . . . hospital work."

5 Bird S. Coler, *Municipal Government* (New York, 1901), pp. 34–35.

6 See City of Brooklyn, *Proceedings of the Board of Aldermen Documents*, vol. 4, document no. 71, pp. 20–21, 1897, for an itemized list of funds distributed. See also Pilcher, "Public Hospitals of Brooklyn," pp. 540–551: "The amount . . . paid is fixed arbitrarily and bears no relation to the amount of work done."

7 Brooklyn, *Proceedings*, p. 20. An asterisk over the name of the Bedford Throat Hospital refers to a note which states that this facility is "probably Brooklyn Throat Hospital."

8 John T. Welles, Bedford Dispensary and Hospital, *Annual Report*, 1898, p. 9.

9 "To Superintendents of Hospitals," *Trained Nurse and Hospital Review*, 20 (Sept. 1895), 160.

10 See Riordan, *Plunkitt of Tammany Hall*, for a contemporary politician's view of reformers and civil service.

11 See William H. Wilson, *Coming of Age: Urban America, 1915–1945* (New York: Wiley, 1974), pp. 58–69, for a brief review of government reforms in the Progressive era city.

12 Riordan, *Plunkitt of Tammany Hall*, p. 19.

13 Ibid., p. 11.

14 See James Weinstein, *The Corporate Ideal in the Liberal State: 1900–1918* (Boston: Beacon Press, 1968), for a review of the interests of the National Association of Manufacturers in state regulation. See also Gabriel Kolko, *The Triumph of Conservatism* (New York: Free Press, 1963); and Samuel Hays, *Conservation and the Gospel of Efficiency: The Progressive Conservation Movement, 1890–1920* (Cambridge, Mass.: Harvard University Press, 1959).

15 Editorial, "The Young Comptroller of New York," *Independent*, 51 (Dec. 28, 1899), 3504.

16 "Bird S. Coler," *NYT*, June 14, 1941, p. 17.

17 See Syrett, *City of Brooklyn*, pp. 266–268, for a brief discussion of the accommodations made. As Syrett illustrates (p. 267), one question raised was: "Is it not dangerous to put in one man's hands, say Richard Croker's, the patronage of the mighty city which is to be formed?"

18 Editorial, "The Young Comptroller," p. 3504.

19 Ibid., p. 3505. See also Bird S. Coler, "Municipal and Business Corruption," *Independent*, 52 (Mar. 15, 1900), 622; and Gustavus Myers, *The History of Tammany Hall* (New York: Dover, 1971), p. 286.

20 State of New York, *Journal of the Senate*, 122nd session, Jan. 1899, p. 433; Charity Organization Society of New York, *18th Annual Report*, July 1899–June 1900, p. 18.

21 Bird S. Coler, "Reform of Public Charity," *Popular Science*, 55 (Oct. 1899), 752.

22 Ibid., p. 753.

23 Charity Organization Society of New York, *18th Annual Report*, July 1899–June 1900, p. 18.

24 Coler, *Municipal Government*, pp. v–vi.

25 Bird S. Coler, "Mistakes of Professional Reformers," *Independent*, 53 (June 20, 1901), 1406–1407.

26 Coler, "Reform of Public Charity," p. 750. See Robert Wiebe, *The Search for Order, 1877–1920* (New York: Hill & Wang, 1967) p. 30, where Wiebe describes some of the effects of technological change on the politics of East Coast cities during the last decades of the nineteenth century: "Then, in the eighties two interrelated factors hastened the first full blown city machines . . . Improvements in urban transit spreading a common malaise and wiping out pockets of political resistance, practically assured control of the city to an organization that could overcome enough local rivalries. Just as this reward dangled, the very scope of the expanding city had so increased the difficulty of providing services that only a central agency could handle them." Though centralization of power aided the bosses, it also aided reformers who controlled important city positions.

27 Coler, "Reform of Public Charity," p. 752.

28 "Private Hospitals," *Charities*, 6 (Jan. 26, 1901), p. 56.

29 Brooklyn Nursery and Infants' Hospital, *29th Annual Report*, June 1900, p. 15.

30 Brooklyn Hospital, *Annual Report*, 1899, p. 8. See also ibid., 1900, p. 8: "The discussion of the city's action . . . has been widespread."

31 Brooklyn Eye and Ear Hospital, *32nd Annual Report*, 1900, p. 6. See also Brooklyn Maternity, *29th Annual Report*, 1899, pp. 9–10: "It is needless to explain that great anxiety has been felt in regard to the future of charitable institutions . . . and what way the distribution of funds for their support may be made or blocked."

32 Methodist Episcopal Hospital, *13th Annual Report*, 1900, p. 15. See Brooklyn

Home for Consumptives, *35th Annual Report*, "Report of the Children's Ward," Oct. 1916, p. 28, for a description of the effects of the policy change on the number of children in the hospital. See also Methodist Episcopal Hospital, *14th Annual Report*, 1901, p. 14: "I regret to report that the City of New York is less liberal with our Hospital than during the previous year"; and Henry W. Maxwell, "Discussion," *BMJ*, 15 (Sept. 1901), 512: "We [at Long Island College Hospital], of course, suffer more or less in the curtailment of public support given to the hospitals and dispensaries in this borough."

33   "Williamsburg: Appeal for Aid," *NYTrib*, Jan. 13, 1903, p. 7.
34   "Williamsburg Hospital Closes," *NYTrib*, Jan. 16, 1903, p. 7.
35   "Hospitals in Need of Aid," *NYTrib*, Oct. 17, 1902, p. 4.
36   Methodist Hospital, *13th Annual Report*, 1900, p. 15.
37   Ibid. See also Brooklyn Maternity, *30th Annual Report*, 1900, pp. 9–10; Brooklyn Hospital, *Annual Report*, 1900, p. 8.
38   "City Subsidies to Private Institutions," Charity Organization Society of New York, *18th Annual Report*, July 1899–June 1900, pp. 18–21. See Roy Lubove, *The Professional Altruist: The Emergence of Social Work as a Career, 1880–1930* (Cambridge, Mass.: Harvard University Press, 1964); and Robert Bremner, *From the Depths: The Discovery of Poverty in the United States* (New York: New York University Press, 1956), for discussion of the Charity Organization Society of New York. Bird S. Coler, in "Abuse of Public Charity," *Popular Science*, 55 (June 1899), 157, also maintained that excessive public contributions would undermine private giving. He hypothesized, however, that public support would tend to decrease in later years, and that there would therefore be a growing need for private giving: "In many cases it happens that when a society begins to receive money from the city private contributions fall off."
39   Jesse T. Duryea, "City versus Independent Hospitals," *BMJ*, 15 (Sept. 1901), 497.
40   "Mr. Simis under Fire," *NYT*, May 16, 1899, p. 3.
41   Duryea, "City versus Independent Hospitals," p. 496. See also "Scope and Support of City Hospitals," *BDE*, Mar. 20, 1901, p. 10 in which Duryea is quoted to the effect that many patients had been found to be able to pay.
42   "Superintendent's Report," Brooklyn Eye and Ear Hospital, *33rd Annual Report*, 1901, pp. 3–4.
43   Brooklyn Eye and Ear Hospital, *34th Annual Report*, 1902, p. 4. See also, for example, idem, *38th Annual Report*, 1906: "Without such valuable assistance the Hospital would be imposed upon oftener than it is"; and idem, *42nd Annual Report*, 1910, p. 11: "As in previous years grateful acknowledgment is due the Brooklyn Bureau of Charities for its willing assistance in investigating these cases."
44   Editorial, "Public Money for Charities," *BMJ*, 13 (Nov. 1899), 698. See also Editorial, "Practical Reform of One Hospital Evil," *BMJ*, 14 (Apr. 1900), 281–282: "The authority to fix the rate of payment to institutions . . . should be a most important help to the city authorities in determining

what the city's future policy will be in reference to the maintenance of its sick poor."

45 Arthur C. Jacobson, "Practical Reform of One Hospital Evil – the System of Inspection Recently Adopted by the Department of Public Charities," *BMJ*, 15 (Sept. 1909), 240. Jacobson continued: "When it comes to medical men attempting to accomplish anything in the way of reform of existing medical evils there is nearly always presented the spectacle of a body wandering in the desert of disorganization."

46 Coler, "Abuse of Public Charity," p. 160.

47 Coler, "Reform of Public Charity," pp. 750–751.

48 See Wiebe, *Search for Order*, p. 169: "Whatever the referencer's specialty, his program relies ultimately upon administration."

49 See also Franklin H. Giddings, "Public Charity and Private Vigilance," *Popular Science*, 55 (Aug. 1899), 433–447. In this reply to Coler's series of papers on reform, Giddings, the well-known sociologist from Columbia University, took issue with the idea that salaries were an inappropriate use of city funds. Giddings, reflecting an older charity view, submitted that charity funds should never be given directly to the poor, but should be spent only on indirect administrative expenses. Direct aid, Giddings held, merely demoralized and debased individual initiative.

50 Pilcher, "Public Hospitals of Brooklyn," p. 539.

51 See Coler, "Abuse of Public Charity," p. 157; idem, *Municipal Government*, pp. 27–28; and idem, "The Subsidy Problem in New York City," *Independent*, 53 (Sept. 12, 1901), 2163.

52 Coler, "Reform of Public Charity," p. 754. See also idem, "Abuse of Public Charity," p. 157; idem, "The Subsidy Problem," p. 2163; and idem, *Municipal Government*, pp. 81–83.

53 Coler, *Municipal Government*, p. 82.

54 Coler, "Reform of Public Charity," pp. 753–755, 757. In this article Coler continued by claiming that there would be "a steady reduction of expenditures for charitable work . . . for several years to come."

55 Duryea, "City versus Independent Hospitals," p. 498: In 1899 the city distributed $175,264 in Brooklyn and Queens; $124,729 was disbursed in 1900.

56 "Scope and Support of City Hospitals," p. 10. See also Duryea, "City versus Independent Hospitals," p. 498: "Five private hospitals . . . discontinued taking public patients."

6. Consolidating control over the small dispensary

1 State Board of Charities, *31st Annual Report*, 1897, Text, Appended Papers, V.I: "Report on the Condition of the Dispensaries of the State of New York," 1897, pp. 617–654. It is impossible to determine the exact number of dispensaries at any one moment, because there was no formal means of registration. Even the state report fails to determine the exact number.

2 State Board of Charities, "Report on the Condition of the Dispensaries," p. 629.

3 See Bushwick and East Brooklyn Dispensary, *12th Annual Report*, 1889–1890, p. 10, for a description of lack of philanthropic support: "We have not annoyed people with appeals"; and Brooklyn Central Dispensary, *33rd Annual Report*, 1888, p. 9: "No bequests . . . and no large private donations have ever reached our treasury." See also Central Dispensary, *36th Annual Report*, 1892, pp. 8–9.

4 Charles Rosenberg, "Social Class and Medical Care in Nineteenth Century America: The Rise and Fall of the Dispensary," *Journal of the History of Medicine*, 29 (Jan. 1974), 32–54.

5 Emmet D. Page, "The Dispensaries of Brooklyn," *BMJ*, 2 (Nov. 1888), 373–374. See also "To Inspect Charities," *NYT*, July 17, 1896, p. 9; "Too Many Dispensaries," *NYT*, July 19, 1896, wherein the reasons for dispensary growth are enumerated; and "Dispensary Relief," *NYT*, June 13, 1897, p. 18. According to the Bushwick and East Brooklyn Dispensary's *19th Annual Report*, May 1897, p. 11, "There is no questioning . . . the fact that the privileges of the Dispensary are abused by a large class of people, who instead of paying the Doctor a fee for his services, prefer to spend their earnings in personal gratification."

6 Page, "The Dispensaries of Brooklyn," pp. 374–376.

7 Ibid., p. 375. See also F. S. Kennedy, "Dispensary Experiences," *BMJ*, 14 (May 1900), 328; and Arthur Bush, "Discussion of Kennedy Paper," *BMJ*, 14 (May 1900), 332: "We know very well, that certain ones have attempted to use the dispensaries as practical feeders."

8 Editorial, "The Abuse of Charity," *BMJ*, 3 (May 1889), 194.

9 Rosenberg, "Social Class and Medical Care," pp. 32–54.

10 Bushwick and East Brooklyn Dispensary, *3rd Annual Report*, 1881, p. 9.

11 Brooklyn Central Dispensary, *33rd Annual Report*, Jan. 1899.

12 Brooklyn Eastern District Dispensary and Hospital, *41st Annual Report*, 1892, pp. 12–13. See also Brooklyn Central Dispensary, *50th Annual Report*, 1906, p. 9.

13 Louis F. Criado, "Our Dispensaries, Hospitals, Philanthropy Frauds, and the Necessity of Medical Reform," *BMJ*, 7 (June 1893), 371.

14 Brooklyn Eastern District Dispensary and Hospital, *40th Annual Report*, 1891, p. 13; Editorial, "Brooklyn Eastern District Dispensary," *BMJ*, 6 (June 1892), 378.

15 Editorial, "Brooklyn Eastern District Dispensary," p. 278. The by-laws listed in the *1st Annual Report* of the Brooklyn Dispensary for Nose, Throat and Lung, 1889, inside cover, included this provision: "Sec. 19. All persons whatsoever shall be admitted to the privileges of the Dispensary for treatment provided, however, that the Surgeon-in-Chief shall be authorized, upon being satisfied that the applicant is able himself, or through his family, to secure proper treatment elsewhere, or for other sufficient cause, to refuse to treat such applicant."

16 Bushwick and East Brooklyn Dispensary, *12th Annual Report*, 1889–1890, p.

15. Throughout the Progressive period, dispensaries' trustees complained about the inconsistent attendance of dispensary physicians. See Northeastern Dispensary, *Minutes*, May 15, 1916, n.p.: "The time of arrival and the average time of service . . . showed up very poorly. On motion . . . the report was accepted with instructions that the Secretary write a letter to the House Physician and report in writing to the Secretary on the unsatisfactory record of some physicians." See also Bushwick and East Brooklyn Dispensary, *13th Annual Report*, May 1891, p. 17: "The Staff has endeavored, in the face of much personal discomfort and sacrifice, by reason of great pressure of private work, to discharge their obligations to the best of their ability"; idem, *18th Annual Report*, May 1896; and idem, *20th Annual Report*, May 1898, p. 10: "The resignation of Dr. James S. King [is regretted] . . . his private practice and his connection with the Bushwick Hospital made it impossible for him to give so much of his time to us."

17   Bushwick and East Brooklyn Dispensary, *18th Annual Report*, May 1896, p. 11. See also BCD, *Minutes*, May 10, 1897, p. 53.

18   See Brooklyn Central Dispensary, *38th Annual Report*, Jan. 1895; and, for a discussion of the plight of the local practitioner during this period, Gerald E. Markowitz and David K. Rosner, "Doctors in Crisis: Medical Education and Medical Reform during the Progressive Era, 1895–1915," in Susan Reverby and David Rosner (eds.), *Health Care in America: Essays in Social History* (Philadelphia: Temple University Press, 1979). See also "The Dispensary War," *JAMA*, 30 (Feb. 26, 1898), 500; W. P. Howle, "What Is to Become of the Physician," *JAMA*, 30 (Jan. 29, 1898), 274; "The Abuse of Medical Charities," *Medical News* (New York), 71 (Oct. 23, 1897), 534; "Abuse," *Maryland Medical Journal*, 34 (Mar. 21, 1896), 411; "Free Hospital Treatment," *JAMA*, 33 (Nov. 25, 1899), 1373; "Our Prospects as a Profession," *JAMA*, 31 (Oct. 15, 1898), 933; "Dispensary Abuse," *Maryland Medical Journal*, 34 (Nov. 16, 1895), 90; C. Phelps, "Causes of the Decline in Income," *Medical News* (New York), 71 (Oct. 23, 1897), 32; F. Jackson, "The Hospital, The Doctor and the Community," *Medical and Surgical Report*, 76 (Mar. 13, 1897), 330; "The Forgotten Doctor," *Virginia's Medical Semimonthly*, 2 (Sept. 10, 1897), 330; "Hospital Abuse," *JAMA*, 33 (June 29, 1897), 1657–1658; J. A. Chase, "Annual Address," *Atlantic Medical Weekly*, 5 (Apr. 4, 1896), 211; "Dispensary Abuse," *Maryland Medical Journal*, 34 (Apr. 4, 1896), 446–447; Brooklyn Eye and Ear Hospital, *Report of the Special Committee on the Abuse of the Clinic* (New York, 1897), p. 13. According to "Personal," *NYT*, June 21, 1897, p. 6, many abusers were "tax payers who imagine that they have a right . . . to an institution to whose support they contribute."

19   Editorial, "Dispensary Bill," *BMJ*, 12 (Mar. 1898), 159. See also Editorial, "Brooklyn Eye and Ear Hospital and Abuse of Dispensary Privileges," *BMJ*, 11 (July 1897), 485–486; "Discussion of Paper," *BMJ*, 14 (May 1900), 336, which quotes one physician as saying, "The great majority of dispensary patients . . . have got more money than I have"; Editorial, "Brooklyn

Eye and Ear Hospital and Abuse of Dispensary Privileges," p. 486; Page, "The Dispensaries of Brooklyn," p. 376, in which Page maintains that the "power to change this . . . rests in the hands of the physicians and in their hands alone," but then accepts the notion that "measures should be introduced, legislative if necessary," to redefine how dispensaries should function; and George Shrady, "A Propagator of Pauperism: The Dispensary," *Forum*, 23 (June 1897), 430.

20   "Dispensary Law Enforced," *Charities*, 15 (Oct. 21, 1905), 109; Lester D. Volk, "The Dispensary Problem – Abuses and Remedy," *Medical Economist*, 2 (Jan. 1914), 7; Michael Davis, "A Medical Bug Bear," *Medical Record*, 86 (Sept. 12, 1914), 460; "The Free Dispensary Evil," *JAMA*, 46 (Mar. 10, 1906), 725–726; "New York's Dispensary System," *Medical Record*, 67 (Mar. 18, 1905), 421.

21   Bird S. Coler, "Reform of Public Charity," *Popular Science*, 55 (Oct. 1899), 753; idem, "The Subsidy Problem in New York City," *Independent*, 53 (Sept. 12, 1901), 2163.

22   Coler, "The Subsidy Problem," p. 2163.

23   Ibid.

24   Bushwick and East Brooklyn Dispensary, *23rd Annual Report*, May 1901, pp. 13–14; idem, *25th Annual Report*, May 1903, p. 12.

25   Bushwick and East Brooklyn Dispensary, *26th Annual Report*, May 1904, pp. 11–12; idem, *27th Annual Report*, May 1905, p. 12; idem, *28th Annual Report*, May 1906, p. 12; idem, *33rd Annual Report*, May 1911, p. 44.

26   Editorial, "Dispensary Law," *BMJ*, 11 (July 11, 1897), 487. See also, "New Dispensary Bill," *BMJ*, 11 (June 1897), 448–449, for the 1897 bill; and "Scientific Business," *BMJ*, 14 (Feb. 1900), 121, for the membership of the Committee on Dispensary Reform.

27   State Board of Charities, "Report on the Condition of the Dispensaries," pp. 639–641.

28   Ibid., pp. 641–643.

29   Ibid., p. 643; see also State of New York, *Laws of 1894*, ch. 171; *Laws of 1895*, ch. 559; *Laws of 1896*, ch. 546.

30   State Board of Charities, "Report on the Condition of the Dispensaries," p. 644. Other reports on the "dispensary abuse" were also widely read. See Editorial, "Abuse of Medical Charity," *BMJ*, 12 (Nov. 1898), 698–700, in which the following local studies are noted: "Report of the Medical Society of the County of New York of its Committee on the Abuses of Medical Charity," transmitted May 24, 1897; "Final Report of the Same Committee," Dec. 1897; "Abstracts of the Proceedings of the New York State Medical Association," 1897; and "The Attitude of the Medical Society of the State of New York toward the Dispensary and Other Medical Bills That Were Before the Legislature of 1898," by Frank Van Fleet. See also Shrady, "A Propagator of Pauperism," pp. 430–431; Shrady called for "a systematic examination of all who plead poverty."

31   Editorial, "Dispensary Bill," *BMJ*, 11 (June 1897), 408.

32   "Dispensary Bill," *BMJ*, 12 (May 1898), 316–317. See also "An Act to

Amend the State Charity Law Relating to Licensing and Regulation of Dispensaries," *State of New York, Laws of 1899*, vol. 1, pp. 791–793; "The Dispensary Bill," *BMJ*, 12 (Mar. 1898), 186–187, for early versions of the law that was to go into effect; and Editorial, "Abuse of Medical Charity," *BMJ*, 12 (Nov. 1898), 699–700, for a review of a paper by Dr. Van Fleet that objected to the role played by some homeopaths in the securing of legislation.

33 NYH's Correspondence contains a series of letters requesting clarification of the meaning of the Dispensary Law. When it was determined that the law would not affect hospital-based dispensaries, the trustees dropped their opposition. See Correspondence, NYH Board of Governors, 1897–1899, folder: Legal-Law Committee.

34 See State Board of Charities, "Dispensary Rules and Regulations," *BMJ*, 13 (Dec. 1899), 760–763.

35 "The Operation of the Dispensary Law," *Charities*, 6 (May 11, 1901), 408–409. See also Charity Organization Society of New York, *19th Annual Report*, June 1901, pp. 31–32: "It is obvious that the law has accomplished as yet comparatively little in checking whatever abuse of medical charity may exist although indirectly it has, doubtless, accomplished something by calling the attention of Managers to the advisability of inquiry and discrimination."

36 Editorial, "The Working of the Dispensary Law," *BMJ*, 14 (June 1900), 21.

37 Brooklyn Eye and Ear Hospital, *32nd Annual Report*, 1900, pp. 3–4; see also Bushwick and East Brooklyn Dispensary, *22nd Annual Report*, May 1900, p. 13. The next year, however, the Bushwick and East Brooklyn Dispensary reported a decline in attendance: See its *23rd Annual Report*, May 1901, p. 16. See also Charity Organization Society of New York, *19th Annual Report*, June 1901, pp. 31–32.

38 William Buck, "Licensed Dispensaries in New York State," *Charities*, 13 (Jan. 14, 1905), 379–380.

39 Brooklyn Association for the Improvement of the Conditions of the Poor, *51st Annual Report*, 1894, p. 13.

40 Ibid., pp. 13–14.

41 Brooklyn Eastern District Dispensary, "By-Laws," 1880, p. 16.

42 Editorial, "Dispensary Question," *BMJ*, 12 (July 1898), 437.

43 Central Throat Hospital, *Annual Report*, Jan. 1898, p. 5. See also Bushwick and East Brooklyn Dispensary, *19th Annual Report*, May 1897, p. 7; and "Dispensary System of New York City," *NYT*, July 14, 1895, p. 28, in which the *Times* quotes one dispensary official on the difficulty inherent in distinguishing between patients: "It is very difficult, and seems impossible to draw a line . . . It was at one time our custom that no one earning more than $15 a week should be allowed the privileges of the dispensary. If a family consisted of one man, wife and one child, this would be a suitable gauge. Suppose [however] there are nine or ten children. What are you going to do then?" Also see "The Hospital and the Community," *Charities*, 51 (Jan. 26, 1901), 53–54: "Speaking of the abuse of medical charity, Dr.

[William] Osler deprecates lavish and indiscriminate giving but he adds: 'The question arises, who is the deserving person? We are all agreed upon the poor man, but how about the relatively poor, the clerk or mechanic with a large family[?]' "

44 "Dispensary Law Enforced," *Charities*, 15 (Oct. 21, 1905), 109. See also F. S. Kennedy, "Discussion," *BMJ*, 14 (May 1900), 337.

45 BCD, *Minutes*, Mar. 8, 1897, pp. 46–47; ibid., Dec. 13, 1897, p. 65.

46 Ibid., Jan. 11, 1897, p. 42.

47 Ibid., Dec. 31, 1897, p. 72. See other statements about the low cost of these facilities in ibid., Dec. 14, 1896, p. 33; ibid., Feb. 26, 1897, p. 48; ibid., June 15, 1896, pp. 25–26. Income also came to the dispensary in the form of interest on bank accounts, investment in bonds and some stocks, and rent from property owned in the city. See, for example, ibid., Oct. 19, 1896, p. 28, for information on the dispensary's stock holdings in the Oswego and Syracuse Railroad.

48 Ibid., June 15, 1896, p. 25.

49 Ibid., Oct. 19, 1896, p. 29. In this same report, the trustees noted that other doctors were also extremely tardy and inconsiderate. Two doctors resigned, one took a leave of absence, and another was "very irregular."

50 Ibid., Dec. 14, 1896, p. 34.

51 See BCD, *Minutes*, By-laws, Article XII, p. 15; BCD, *Minutes*, Jan. 11, 1897, p. 38, ibid., Dec. 14, 1896, p. 34.

52 BCD, *Minutes*, Jan. 11, 1892, p. 38; ibid., Dec. 13, 1897, p. 65.

53 Ibid., May 17, 1898, p. 85.

54 Ibid., Apr. 9, 1899, p. 144. See also, ibid., Oct. 14, 1901: Three doctors resigned and there were no replacements available.

55 Ibid., Apr. 14, 1902, p. 201.

56 See the report on Length of Service in ibid., n.p. (last page of vol. 1), June 12, 1901.

57 BCD, *Minutes*, Nov. 9, 1896, p. 31.

58 Ibid., Oct. 10, 1898, p. 92.

59 Ibid., Nov. 14, 1898, p. 95.

60 Ibid., p. 98. See also ibid., July 28, 1899, p. 119, for a statement of Comptroller Coler's demand for information concerning the number of cases treated at the dispensary.

61 Ibid., Jan. 8, 1900, p. 132.

62 Ibid., Feb. 12, 1900, p. 135.

63 Ibid., Oct. 23, 1900, p. 156.

64 Ibid., Nov. 12, 1900, p. 155.

65 Ibid., Oct. 23, 1900, p. 156.

66 Ibid., Feb. 7, 1898, p. 75.

67 Ibid., Feb. 14, 1898, p. 76.

68 Ibid., Apr. 11, 1898, p. 83.

69 Ibid., Feb. 12, 1900, p. 135. In Apr. 1900 the board received a communication from the Medical Society of the County of Kings, asking for "uniform enforcement of the Dispensary Law," and the board asked for per-

mission to attend the society's future meetings. See ibid., Apr. 9, 1900.

70 Ibid., Feb. 15, 1900, p. 137.

71 Ibid., Apr. 19, 1900, p. 144.

72 Ibid., Apr. 9, 1900, p. 146.

73 Ibid., pp. 146–147.

74 Ibid., Oct. 23, 1900, p. 156 (letter). The "special committee appointed to consider ways and means for the future reported in favor of a charge of ten cents for each prescription." It was adopted unanimously, "with the exception of Mr. Clark" (ibid., Nov. 12, 1900, p. 155).

75 Ibid., Nov. 12, 1900, p. 155.

76 Ibid., Dec. 10, 1900, p. 158; ibid., Mar. 11, 1901, p. 171; ibid., Jan. 11, 1904, n.p.

77 Ibid., Dec. 14, 1903, p. 235.

78 Ibid., July 14, 1904, p. 268.

79 See the minutes of the dispensary from 1915 to 1920 for a complete account of the continuing crisis.

7. The battle for Morningside Heights

1 Christine Boyer, "Planning the City of Capital" (unpublished manuscript, Columbia University School of Architecture, Department of Urban Planning, 1979). Boyer discusses the ideological foundations of the turn-of-the-century urban planning profession. See also, Elizabeth Blackmar, "Housing and Property Relations in New York City, 1785–1850" (Unpublished dissertation, Harvard University, 1981), for a fascinating account of land-use in an earlier period.

2 NYH, "The financial condition . . . of the Society of New York Hospital," Apr. 17, 1866, p. 1, in Governing Board of NYH, *Reports, Addresses, etc.*, set 1, box 1/2 73D in the hospital's archives. (All references regarding NYH refer to materials in the archives unless otherwise noted.)

3 Ibid., pp. 4–6.

4 Ibid., p. 4.

5 Ibid., pp. 5–6.

6 For a listing of real estate owned by the hospital and income derived from that real estate, see State of New York, *Legislative Record*, 111th session, Albany, May 7, 1888, p. 975, in NYH, *Secretary-Treasurer's Papers*, 1888–1889, box 10 of 68, folder: 1888, Bd. Gov. Papers (hereafter referred to as Bd. Gov. Papers).

7 Charles Lockwood, *Manhattan Moves Uptown* (New York: Houghton Mifflin, 1976), pp. 283–284.

8 Ibid., pp. 314–315.

9 Ibid., pp. 315–317.

10 See "Now for Bloomingdale," *New York World*, Mar. 1888, in Bd. Gov. Papers.

11 "Bloomingdale – Its Great Untaxed Estate," *New York Herald*, Apr. 1888, in Bd. Gov. Papers.

12 "Is It a Charity or Not?" *New York World*, Mar. 5, 1888, in Bd. Gov. Papers.
13 "Bloomingdale – an Incubus – Real Estate Men Declare the Asylum Depreciates Property – a Blight on the West Side," *New York World*, Mar. 18, 1888, in Bd. Gov. Papers.
14 "Hot Shot for Bloomingdale," *New York Herald*, Feb. 9, 1888, in Bd. Gov. Papers.
15 "Bloomingdale – Its Great Untaxed Estate"; "Hot Shot for Bloomingdale."
16 See Census Office, Department of the Interior, *Vital Statistics of New York City and Brooklyn, Covering a Period of Six Years Ending May 31, 1890* (Washington, D.C.: Government Printing Office, 1894), for a detailed description of the health status, national origins, and demographic and socioeconomic characteristics of the area.
17 Ibid., p. 112.
18 Ibid., pp. 157–158.
19 "Bloomingdale – Its Great Untaxed Estate."
20 Henry C. Crane, "History of the Society of New York Hospital, 1769–1920" (microfilm, NYH Archives), p. 376; "Asylum Comm. Governors, Dec. 1866," in Bd. Gov. Papers.
21 See State of New York, Assembly Bill no. 84, Jan. 17, 1888, "An Act to Lay Out and Improve . . . ," in Bd. Gov. Papers.
22 See "Short Cut Across Lots," *New York World*, Mar. 5, 1888, in Bd. Gov. Papers; "Bloomingdale Asylum," *New York Herald*, May 5, 1888, Bd. Gov. Papers; and "Opulent Insane Must Quit," *New York Herald*, Mar. 8, 1888.
23 "Hot Shot for Bloomingdale."
24 See Charles Strong to Elbridge Gerry, Feb. 6, 1888, in Bd. Gov. Papers.
25 "Bloomingdale – Its Great Untaxed Estate"; "Hot Shot for Bloomingdale." In the latter Bixby shows "how the State has given thousands of dollars to Bloomingdale and with what arrogance the poor were turned away and a grip kept on a most commanding site tax free."
26 "Hot Shot for Bloomingdale." See also "Is It a Charity or Not?"; and "Not for the Poor Insane," *World*, Mar. 1888, in Bd. Gov. Papers. The last of these articles states that "property owners in the twelfth ward hope that the bill which has just been introduced . . . will meet with a better fate than similar measures."
27 "Bloomingdale Asylum," *New York Evening Post*, Mar. 1888; "Bloomingdale Must Go," *New York World*, Mar. 11, 1888; "Money in Lunatics," *New York World*, Mar. 1888; "Now for Bloomingdale," *New York World*, Mar. 1888; "Shelled by Their Own Guns," *New York World*, Mar. 25, 1888; "Bloomingdale Asylum," *NYTrib*, Mar. 25, 1888 – all in Bd. Gov. Papers.
28 "Not for the Poor Insane."
29 "Threatening the Asylum Board," *New York World*, Mar. 22, 1888, in Bd. Gov. Papers.
30 "Bloomingdale – an Incubus."
31 "Bloomingdale Must Go"; "Now for Bloomingdale."
32 "Should It Be Exempt?" *New York Star*, Mar. 10, 1888, in Bd. Gov. Papers.
33 See telegram from Gerry to James Husted, Republican from Peekskill,

whom Gerry told to "refer Connelly's bill . . . to Ways and Means," in Bd. Gov. Papers. See also State of New York, *Legislative Record*, 111th session, Albany, May 7, 1883, p. 969.

34 "Bloomingdale Asylum," *New York Evening Post*, Mar. 1888, in Bd. Gov. Papers.

35 State of New York, *Legislative Record*, 111th session, Albany, May 7, 1888, p. 972.

36 See the Report of the Senate Committee on Taxation, in State of New York, *Legislative Record*, 111th session, Albany, May 7, 1888, pp. 969–976; see also "A Victory for the Bloomingdales," *New York World*, May 5(?), 1888; and "Bloomingdale Asylum," *New York Herald*, May 5, 1888, in Bd. Gov. Papers.

37 Charles Strong to Elbridge Gerry, May 5, 1888, in Bd. Gov. Papers.

38 See various letters in Bd. Gov. Papers for descriptions of Bliss's increasing activity in Albany. Also see the short note on Bliss in *Who's Who in America*, vol. 1, *1897–1942*, p. 107.

39 Press clippings, n.d., in NYH Papers, 1888–1889, folder: 1889 Law Committee Papers. See also Ernest Hornsby to Elbridge Gerry, Jan. 25, 1889, in NYH Papers, 1888–1889, folder: 1889 Law Committee Papers; and undated newspaper clipping in NYH Papers, 1888–1889, folder: 1889 Law Committee Papers: "Mr. Crosby was the only city member who voted No."

40 Ernest Hornsby to Elbridge Gerry, Jan. 25, 1889, in NYH Papers, 1888–1889, folder: 1889 Law Committee Papers. See State of New York, Senate bill no. 78, Jan. 22, 1889, "An Act to Authorize the Street Opening . . ."; and Senate Bill no. 79, Jan. 22, 1889, "An Act to Provide for Assessment and Taxation . . ." – both in NYH Papers, 1888–1889, folder: 1889 Law Committee Papers.

41 See State of New York, Assembly Bill no. 790, Jan. 10, 1889, "An Act . . . to exempt Property . . ."; and Assembly Bill no. 70, Jan. 10, 1889, "An Act to Lay Out and Improve One Hundred and Sixteenth Street" – both in NYH Papers, 1888–1889, folder: 1889 Law Committee Papers.

42 See, for example, the notices announcing the sale of hospital property in NYH Papers, 1888–1889, folder: Real Estate Committee.

43 Charles Strong to Elbridge Gerry, Dec. 19, 1888, in NYH Papers, 1888–1889, folder: 1889 Law Committee Papers. The two petitions are also in this folder, as is a letter from Charles Nichols to James Brown, Feb. 7, 1889, in which Nichols reports that the petition was delivered to the assemblyman from White Plains and that it contained the signatures of the president of the council of White Plains and of five of the town's six trustees.

44 Charles Nichols to James Brown, Feb. 7, 1889, in NYH Papers, 1888–1889, folder: 1889 Law Committee Papers. By Mar. 1889, the governors were receiving extremely anxious queries from a number of people, including Nichols. One such letter shows Nichols as clearly worried that the lobbying effort in Albany is failing: "I asked . . . Mrs. Judge Ferris . . . to see

[one of the hospital's supporters in the legislature] and set him right in regard to the purposes of the Governors with respect to removing from Bloomingdale to the country." See Nichols to Gerry, Mar. 7, 1889, and Mrs. Judge Ferris to Nichols (copy), n.d. (in which Mrs. Ferris says that she is worried that the "case has not been in good hands") – both in NYH Papers, 1888–1889, folder: 1889 Law Committee Papers.

45 Elbridge Gerry to James M. Brown, May 17, 1889, in NYH Papers, 1888–1889, folder: 1889 Law Committee Papers.

46 See ibid., Elbridge T. Gerry to Cornelius N. Bliss, June 7, 1889, in NYH Papers, 1888–1889, folder: 1889 Law Committee Papers; and undated newspaper clippings in Bd. Gov. Papers, in which the compromise nature of the passage of these two bills is recognized and discussed.

47 See Who's Who in America, vol. 1, 1897–1942, s.v. "Gerry, Elbridge."

48 See this extremely informative document: "Declaration of the Society of New York Hospital Restricting Real Estate," Mar. 19, 1889, in NYH Papers, 1888–1889, folder: 1889 Law Committee Papers. In this covenant, the Hospital not only commits itself to these restrictions, but commits the buyer not to sell to anyone who would break the covenant: "And the said Society doth hereby covenant to and with the purchasers above described, that all of the tracts . . . shall be conveyed subject to the covenant and restrictions herein contained."

49 "Declaration of the Society of the New York Hospital Restricting Real Estate."

50 Seth Low to H. H. Cammann, Nov. 13, 1891, in NYH Papers, 1890–1893, folder: 1891 Sundry Papers and Letters, folder 1.

51 Ibid.

52 Columbia College, "Statement of the Committee on Site," Jan. 1892, in NYH Papers, 1890–1893, folder: 1892 Exec. Committee.

53 Martin J. Schiesl, The Politics of Efficiency: Municipal Administration and Reform in America, 1888–1920 (Berkeley and Los Angeles: University of California Press, 1977), pp. 18–20.

54 See ibid., for a more detailed analysis of Low's views.

55 See Thomas Fulton to Cornelius Bliss, Mar. 22, 1899, in which the support of the hospital for the fight is requested; and the financial statement of the Amsterdam Avenue Defense Committee, Aug. 1899, in which it is shown that the largest single contributors to the committee, all of whom gave between $500 and $1,000, were J. J. Astor, William Astor, Columbia College, St. John the Divine, New York Hospital, and the West End Association; both documents are in NYH Papers, 1898–1899, folder: 1899 Real Estate.

56 Schiesl, The Politics of Efficiency, pp. 32–33. Schiesl also gives important information on the origins of the reform and efficiency movements; he sees the later progressive movement as a reflection of the class bias of displaced patricians and middle-class groups.

57 See Schiesl, The Politics of Efficiency, for a detailed account of this effort.

8. Looking backward

1   See "Brooklyn's Oldest Hospital Built Anew," *Modern Hospital*, 7 (Nov. 1916), 661–666. The engraving on the first page of this article was reproduced on a publicity brochure published by the hospital in the same year.

Select bibliography

Books

Ashley, Jo Ann. *Hospitals, Paternalism, and the Role of the Nurse* (New York: Teachers College Press, 1976).

Bremner, Robert H. *From the Depths: The Discovery of Poverty in the United States* (New York: New York University Press, 1956).

Brieger, Gert, *Medical America in the Nineteenth Century* (Baltimore: Johns Hopkins University Press, 1972).

Burrow, James G. *AMA: Voice of American Medicine* (Baltimore: Johns Hopkins Press, 1963).

Duffy, John. *A History of Public Health in New York City, 1866–1966* (New York: Russell Sage Foundation, 1974).

Duffy, John. *The Healers: The Rise of the Medical Establishment* (New York: McGraw-Hill, 1976).

Hirsh, Joseph. *Saturday, Sunday and Everyday: The History of the United Hospital Fund of New York* (New York: United Hospital Fund, 1954).

Kett, Joseph. *The Formation of the American Medical Profession: The Role of Institutions, 1760–1860* (New Haven: Yale University Press, 1968).

Levitan, Tina. *Islands of Compassion: A History of the Jewish Hospitals of New York* (New York: T. Wayne, 1964).

Lubove, Roy. *The Professional Altruist: The Emergence of Social Work as a Career, 1880–1930* (Cambridge, Mass.: Harvard University Press, 1965).

Pernick, Martin S. *A Calculus of Suffering: Pain and Anesthesia in Nineteenth Century Medicine* (New York: Columbia University Press, forthcoming).

Reverby, Susan, and David Rosner (eds.). *Health Care in America: Essays in Social History* (Philadelphia: Temple University Press, 1979).

Reverby, Susan. " 'Apprenticeship to Duty': The Rationalization of American Nursing, 1869–1940" (Ph.D. dissertation, Boston University, 1982).

Rosen, George. *The Specialization of Medicine, with Particular Reference to Ophthalmology* (New York: Froben, 1944).

Rosenberg, Charles E. *The Cholera Years: The United States in 1832, 1849 and 1866* (Chicago: University of Chicago Press, 1962).

Rosenberg, Charles E. (ed.) *Healing and History: Essays for George Rosen* (New York: Science History, 1979).

Rosenkrantz, Barbara G. *Public Health and the State: Changing Views in Massachusetts, 1842–1936* (Cambridge, Mass.: Harvard University Press, 1972).

Rothman, David. *The Discovery of the Asylum* (Boston: Little, Brown, 1971).

Rothstein, William G. *American Physicians in the 19th Century from Sects to Science* (Baltimore: Johns Hopkins University Press, 1972).

Schneider, David, and Albert Deutsch. *History of Public Welfare in New York State, 1867–1940* (Chicago: University of Chicago Press, 1941).

Shyrock, Richard H. *Medicine and Society in America: 1660–1860* (New York: New York University Press, 1960).

Starr, Paul. *The Transformation of American Medicine* (New York: Basic, 1982).

Stevens, Rosemary. *American Medicine and the Public Interest* (New Haven: Yale University Press, 1971).

Vogel, Morris J. *The Invention of the Modern Hospital: Boston, 1870–1930* (Chicago: University of Chicago Press, 1980).

Vogel, Morris J., and Charles E. Rosenberg (eds.). *The Therapeutic Revolution: Essays in the Social History of American Medicine* (Philadelphia: University of Pennsylvania Press, 1979).

Articles

Kunitz, Stephen J. "Efficiency and Reform in the Financing and Organization of American Medicine in the Progressive Era," *Bulletin of the History of Medicine* 55 (Winter 1981), 497–515.

Markowitz, Gerald E., and David K. Rosner. "Doctors in Crisis: Medical Education and Medical Reform during the Progressive Era, 1895–1915," in Susan Reverby and David Rosner (eds.), *Health Care in America: Essays in Social History* (Philadelphia: Temple University Press, 1979), pp. 185–205.

Maynard, Edwin P., Jr. "The Practice of Medicine in 1921," *Bulletin of the New York Academy of Medicine*, 48 (July 1972), 807–817.

Reverby, Susan. "Stealing the Golden Eggs: Ernest Amory Codman and the Science and Management of Medicine," *Bulletin of the History of Medicine*, 55 (Summer 1981), 156–171.

Rosen, George. "The Hospital: Historical Sociology of a Community Institution," in George Rosen, *From Medical Police to Social Medicine* (New York: Science History, 1974), pp. 274–303.

Rosenberg, Charles E. "And Heal the Sick: The Hospital and Patient in Nineteenth Century America," *Journal of Social History*, 10 (June 1977), 428–447.

Rosenberg, Charles E. "Social Class and Medical Care in Nineteenth Century America: The Rise and Fall of the Dispensary," *Journal of the History of Medicine*, 29 (Jan. 1974), 32–54.

Rosner, David. "Gaining Control: Reform, Reimbursement and Politics in New York's Community Hospitals, 1890–1915," *American Journal of Public Health*, 70 (May 1980), 533–542.

Rosner, David. "Business at the Bedside: Health Care in Brooklyn, 1895–1915," in Susan Reverby and David Rosner (eds.), *Health Care in America: Essays in Social History* (Philadelphia: Temple University Press, 1979), pp. 117–131.

Sigerist, Henry E. "An Outline of the Development of the Hospital," *Bulletin of the Institute of the History of Medicine*, 4 (July 1936), 573–581.

Vogel, Morris J. "Patrons, Practitioners, and Patients: The Voluntary Hospital in Mid-Victorian Boston," in Daniel Walker Howe (ed.), *Victorian America* (Philadelphia: University of Pennsylvania Press, 1976), pp. 121–138.

Index